($895 NEW)

TRANSFORMATION AND IDENTITY

TRANSFORMATION AND IDENTITY

The Face and Plastic Surgery

Frances Cooke Macgregor

WITH AN INTRODUCTION BY *Margaret Mead*

AND FOREWORD BY *John Marquis Converse*

Quadrangle / The New York Times Book Company

DESIGNED BY VINCENT TORRE

Library of Congress Cataloging in Publication Data

Macgregor, Frances M   Cooke
    Transformation and identity.

    Bibliography: p.
    1. Face—Abnormities and deformities—Psychological
aspects. 2. Surgery, Plastic. I. Title.
[DNLM: 1. Face—Abnormalities. 2. Face—Surgery.
3. Identification (Psychology). 4. Surgery, Plastic.
WE705 M147t]
RD763.M32 1974   617'.52   74-77943
ISBN 0-8129-0478-8

Contents

Chapter Six
Surgery: The Patient and the Surgeon

Chapter Seven
Some Dilemmas of Cosmetic Surgery

Chapter Eight
Potential Lost and Potential Realized

Introduction

In studies of human behavior, the student is hampered by being of the same species as those whose career lines are to be studied. Unlike the geneticist, to whom the fruit flies provide a new generation every week, or the astronomer, whose stars abide in their courses, those of us who study human beings can only live as long and run as fast and stay awake as long as those we study. Furthermore, the human sciences are so young that most of us have had no body of theory or practice to fall back upon. Plastic surgery is a young practice, and the social psychological studies of disfigurement and rehabilitation are young sciences. We are all the more fortunate, therefore, to have in this book the record of a quarter of a century of association between Frances Macgregor, pioneer in studies of the social accompaniments of disfigurement and reconstructive surgery, and John Marquis Converse, a leading innovator in the field of plastic surgery. Because of their long collaboration, Frances Macgregor has been able to follow the subsequent fate of those whose extreme birth defects were corrected in childhood and those who were injured in adulthood. Instead of prognostications about what would happen to a child born with a malformed face or a beautiful woman maimed almost beyond recognition, we have in this book an account of what *did* happen. In the human sciences, there are so many factors to consider that prophesies often prove empty, and retrospective studies become our major path to understanding. But too often these reconstructions involve a past for which we have no firm data. Not so in this book. The human beings described here were well known, first as patients, and later as friendly collaborators who were willing to relate to Frances Macgregor what the vicissitudes of their lives had been.

It is one of the comforting features of our times—times in which so many new dangers and terrors challenge the meaning of human existence—that as our knowledge and ability to alleviate some of the burdens that humankind has borne through the ages grow, so also our compassion grows. As we begin to develop ways of remedying birth defects and accidental injuries that once had to be sustained without hope, we can afford to look at the victims, and to look at the fortunate—the undisfigured who have in the past been unable to bear to look at those who represent their own fears and repulsions. The mother of a child with a harelip once had no recourse except to wring her hands and weep: "Was it my fault? Was it the fault of the hare that crossed my path?" The husband, whose error while driving has resulted in an accident that marred his wife's face forever, could only seek to atone—and perhaps receive her scorn—or flee from the face that he no longer recognized. People in primitive villages often sought to include the disfigured and the crippled who survived neglect and rejection by making them the butt of jokes, which (though cruel) nevertheless treated them as human. But in the great anonymous urban societies of the present day, most people have turned away, refused to empathize or to deal with the disfigured for whose disfigurement they felt nothing could be done. Compassion was frozen in the powerlessness of the spectators.

But as plastic surgery developed into a more and more precise and delicate practice—as whole faces were reconstructed, and those who would once have been hopelessly disfigured returned to a fuller and more dignified participation in society—compassion could grow, and with it, social science enquiries into the consequences of facial disfigurement. It is a notable feature of the mental health professions (and those parts of the social sciences that have become essential components of mental health) that they have developed from the combination of compassion and newly acquired ability to help the unfortunate and the stigmatized.

From this combination of skill in diagnosis and treatment, compassion that could now be more freely expressed, and the development of psychological and cultural theory comes a new respect for those who have to cope with various kinds of disfigurement, a respect that in the past was smothered beneath a sense of impotence, rage, and fear.

Frances Macgregor's sociological work has been interrelated with her ethnographic photography, studies of American Indians, the book that she and I did together (*Growth and Culture, A Photographic Study of Balinese Childhood*), and her experience as a medical photographer. From her hospital studies, she developed an interest in the responses of members of different cultures to disfigurement. Exploring the plight of the disfigured (the ways in which societies stigmatized, avoided, or ignored their condition, attributed it to black magic, ancestral curses, the punishment of God) led her to those who were practicing the amelioration of these conditions. And as she studied the individual patient and his family seeking relief from a terrible accident, she included the responses, real and imagined, of others to the patients she interviewed. So she built up, from observations of the patients themselves and from her work with the physicians, nurses, and social workers, an understanding of their responses to disfigurement. This book, then, includes us all: the disfigured to whom modern surgical skills are giving back a place in society, those who work directly with them, their employers and friends and relatives, and the great anonymous crowd that has passed by, shuddering, on the other side.

But it is important, I believe, to realize certain things about American cultural attitudes that are particularly relevant to our reactions toward any sort of defect. We are taught as children that we should not stare, should not ask questions, should not, in fact, direct any kind of attention at all toward someone who is crippled or disfigured in any way. This teaching is done in the name of compassion. But, by that very compassion, we have excluded the disfigured and crippled from full participation, sometimes even to the point of slamming a door on someone on crutches coming through that door behind us. Any deficiency, any handicap, any defect that could not be remedied, had to be ignored to the point of ostracism.

But once there is a possibility that the defect can be reduced or minimized or compensated for, our attitude changes from one of painful inattention to active concern. Something should be done; cripples should have prostheses, paraplegics should have special cars they can drive, the congenitally disfigured and those mutilated in accidents or by disease should have plastic surgery. Whatever is wrong that can be fixed, should be fixed. So, as plastic surgeons become more skilled, as more of those who once would have had to go through life in unrelieved despair are rehabilitated, new problems arise. Those who know that something can be done are freer to say something ought to be done. And those who know that something has been done are freer to respond with curiosity and concern. Those disabled Americans who have learned to move easily among others, in wheelchairs, blind, with cunning hooks for hands, have learned that if they take the initiative, and articulately explain their state, others are able to respond with empathy and interest. But these responses often take the form of questions: "How do you work those hooks?" "How do you get across a street?" "How do you get out of that wheelchair at night?" Questions that would once have been avoided are now asked easily. But questioning, active curiosity, is the device that Americans use to relate to anyone toward whom they may otherwise have to appear to be indifferent, agonizingly turning their eyes away.

Plastic surgery is too new, the intricacies of its practice are still too specialized, the complications introduced by cosmetic surgery to hide age or ethnic identity or imputed identity too embarrassing for the average person to be able to deal with reconstructed faces as easily as he deals with substitute arms and legs, glass eyes, hearing aids, and the white canes of the blind. This is a transition period. More and more people have experienced what plastic surgery can do and have begun to approach the birth-injured child or the victim of an accident with hope, optimistic advice, admonishment toward constructive action. But for those who have lived many years as the parents of a congenitally imperfect child, as sibling or spouse or child of someone injured in adulthood, quivering in shame and anger over the looks in other peoples' eyes, these new, curious, articulate approaches seem pitiless and intrusive. And for the person who has experienced virtual extrusion from the human race, it is not easy to re-enter it by way of questions: "Was that a burn or a birthmark?" "Did your child have a true cleft palate?" Yet this is surely the next step. As we come to realize the dynamics of injury, and the ways in which members of a particular culture respond (especially to the face, which is in fact the interface between private person and public life), some modus vivendi must be established. If the reconstructed person is to be a full member of society, then he (or she) must take his place, with acceptance of his full individuality (just as this is necessary for those previously excluded because of color or sex or age), acknowledge with dignity who he is, and expect neither fear nor favor. In the case of the crippled or the blind or the aged, relationships can be established by help being requested, and directed, by the person who needs help or who feels that other people have a need to give help. But for those who wish to relate to the facially disfigured there is no easy substitute for the kind of help that can be offered to someone on crutches. There is no other activity that can be eagerly, perhaps even officiously, substituted for face-to-face contact, because, for the facially disfigured, it is only face-to-face contact that will suffice to accord them full humanity.

This means, in practice, that we not only need support for reconstructive surgery, counseling, and supporting care for all those who are disfigured, but that we need practice (for the great mass of those who have intact though not necessarily beautiful faces) in looking directly and straightforwardly into the faces of the disfigured. This is the point where the borderline between reconstructive surgery and cosmetic surgery exists. There is no research to substantiate this, but I suspect that those who are most repelled by the disfigured are those who are also most dissatisfied with their own faces, those to whom very small and almost imperceptible defects loom disproportionately large. It is true that those nose.

who have been dowered with beauty may feel a passionate sense of the unfairness of life when they encounter someone who has had the opposite fate. But such a natural dowry, if it is fully appreciated, brings generosity. Not so, the exaggerated rejection of some small defect, some weakness of chin, or slightly slanted

It is here that one may argue for the importance of cosmetic surgery as well as reconstructive surgery, trivial as it may often seem, as a demand on the time of the skilled surgeon who can only operate so many hours a day. The fewer members of the public there are who shudder away from the reflections of their own very moderately displeasing or unfashionable faces, the easier it will be to build a climate of opinion within which those with reconstructed faces may move with a full sense of identity. Today, we accord this full identity only to the blind, whose courage and insistence upon playing as normal a role as possible evoke responsive admiration and recognition from the sighted. This book, with its poignant records of suffering and of the extraordinary courage of those who have fought their way through to economic self-sufficiency and social participation, should do much to increase our capacity to accept and receive those whose faces still bear the marks of the injury that no amount of plastic surgical skill can completely remove.

There is much loose talk today about the coldness, the impersonality, the exploitative nature of the social sciences—some deserved, some undeserved. On the contrary, sociology has often been discounted in those respects in which it has developed from the compassion and the passion of those who rebelled against social conditions that produce unnecessary suffering. There is sometimes even a very close connection between an insistence on rigor, on statistics, on experimental design, and such a deep anger at the human condition that it must be overlaid and concealed at all costs. In many studies of stigma, of discrimination, and of despair, the human element seems to be lacking. But in Frances Macgregor's case this is not so. Meticulous attention to recording her long, intensive interviews, meticulous preservation of relevant social and cultural detail, and cooperative work with clinical psychologists and psychiatrists and with the operating surgeons make her work sound and objective. But this is done without in any way masking or detracting from her genuine, unashamed concern for the suffering she has witnessed and recorded. For this we should be very grateful.

Margaret Mead
American Museum of Natural History
New York City 1974

Foreword

The problems posed by facial disfigurement in our society are not only those of reconstructive plastic surgery and physical restoration but those that directly concern the mental health of the patient, his family, and his community. These facts were impressed upon me during the early part of World War II when I operated upon some of the pilots of the Royal Air Force who had sustained severe facial wounds. Because of the multiple stages and the prolonged periods that were frequently required for their treatment, I became friendly with these men and learned about some of their nonsomatic problems. They were young, they were heroes, and were in full possession of their mental and physical strength; people were proud of them and proud to be seen with them. When it came to more intimate relations, however, certain barriers appeared—the repulsion evoked by a disfigured face. One young officer said, "When I take a girl out to dinner, all goes well until I kiss her—I can then feel her shudder."

On my return from World War II, through the intermediary of a mutual friend, I was privileged to meet Frances Cooke Macgregor, a social scientist who began to interview my patients. Following her exploratory research we were able to conduct the first interdisciplinary study on the social and psychological implications of facial deformities, through a grant from the National Institute of Mental Health.

The number of individuals with severe facial disfigurement is far larger than is generally realized by the public. Disfigured persons are less accepted in our society than are those with other types of physical disabilities, and are therefore more reluctant to appear in public.

Unfortunately, the number of disfigured persons increases daily, with industrial and traffic accidents, war injuries, disease, and criminal assaults contributing to the growing total. The National Academy of Science reports (*The New York Times*, Sept. 11, 1972) that each year 52 million Americans suffer injury. Although no specific figures are available, the number of injuries to the face, exposed and unprotected as it is, may be assumed to be very high.

Burns alone account for approximately 2 million injuries a year (explosions, flammable clothing, etc.) according to the National Health Survey data. Although the extent of the injuries may vary, a high proportion of burn victims sustain injuries that are permanent and incapacitating.

Other causes of facial disfigurements, aside from accidents, are those surgically induced as a result of cancer and those caused by radiation procedures.

Birth defects also account for a substantial number of facial deformities. It has been estimated that in 1 birth in 16 a baby is born with some type of congenital defect, ranging from a small mole to a serious heart deficiency, whereas 1 child in 700 is born with a cleft lip and/or palate.

In the minds of the public as well as in many of those in the health professions, plastic surgery and cosmetic surgery are synonymous. In an informal survey conducted among physicians (nonsurgeons) as to what first came to mind when plastic surgery was mentioned, the majority of responses were "cosmetic surgery" and "high fees." In the last few years we have seen a plethora of books, newspaper and magazine articles, and television shows devoted to the subject of cosmetic surgery, with emphasis on face lifts, correction of baggy eyes and double chins, and so forth, that can help people look more youthful and attractive. These corrective procedures are often of considerable psychological import for the patient. Overlooked or not fully realized, however, are the thousands of reconstructive surgical procedures performed in the United States by plastic surgeons to eradicate or ameliorate severe malformations or disfigurements that otherwise could mean social and psychological death for the victim.

Because the spotlight has largely been on the cosmetic aspects, comparatively little attention has been given to the scientific study of the sociological and psychological consequences of conspicuous facial deviance and the attendant problems of adjustment, management, and rehabilitation. This book is evidence of the research efforts that have been and are being directed along this line. Clearly demonstrated is the fact that in plastic surgery, no less than in other areas of medicine, the surgical services, as well as the social and vocational rehabilitation services, must include both an awareness and application of the social, psychological, and cultural dimensions that have relevance for the understanding and total rehabilitation of the patient.

Plastic surgery performed as early as possible where it can correct or improve a congenital anomaly or facial injury is essential in order to prevent deep and permanent psychic wounds. Where surgery can accomplish only partial correction or none at all, psychotherapy—techniques that are far from perfected at present —may help patients adjust to their predicament. Those who have endured long periods of disfigurement resulting in a disturbance of the personality and the sense of identity stand in particular need of psychological assistance. But the problem of disfigurement is not that of the victim alone, as the testimony of those described in this book demonstrates. It is the nonhandicapped who by their negative and prejudicial attitudes help create and then perpetuate the handicap itself and the consequent burden of suffering.

John Marquis Converse, M.D.,
Lawrence D. Bell Professor of Plastic Surgery,
New York University School of Medicine;
Director of the Institute of
Reconstructive Plastic Surgery,
New York University Medical Center
New York City 1974

Preface

Facial disfigurement is one of man's gravest handicaps. Wearing his defect on his face, he suffers from the highest visibility. As studies have shown, esthetic rejection is the most frequently reported basis for feelings of aversion, and rejection of those whose faces are marred is even greater than that of amputees, the blind, or the deaf. Indeed problems of employability and social intercourse are of such magnitude that many disfigured persons remain in seclusion. In sum, the problems of the facially handicapped are social and psychological and lie squarely in the area of mental health.

This book is a synthesis of my research and writings on the social, psychological, and cultural implications of facial deviations and plastic surgery, ranging from severe to slight, in which I have been engaged directly or peripherally for more than twenty years. Its purpose is to make a definitive statement of this field as a subspecialty of the social psychology of the handicapped, to deal with its major areas and subdivisions, to delineate the problems, and to suggest, largely by implication, approaches for management and rehabilitation as well as areas for future research. While each section considers the problem from a different perspective, the unifying thread is the significance of appearance in personality formation, social interaction, and identity.

The research reported here was done mainly at the following institutions: the New York University School of Medicine, the Manhattan Eye, Ear and Throat Hospital and the Institute of Reconstructive Plastic Surgery, New York University Medical Center.

In the course of the research I have interviewed both pre- and postoperatively hundreds of patients and their families, and observed them in hospitals and private offices, in reception rooms, and at evaluation conferences. I have attended patients' operations, visited them in their hospital rooms, and accompanied them in public places. Interviews were nondirective and, for most of the studies reported in this book, interview hours per person ranged in general from four to thirty. Very fortunately, I have been able to follow and make longitudinal studies of a number of patients over a period of years—in some cases twenty or more. For specific projects, sentence completion tests and self-evaluation scales were used. Patients were informed of the research nature of our work and with their knowledge I took verbatim notes or used a tape recorder. In all reports I have taken care to protect the privacy of individuals and their families by disguising their identity but at the same time preserving relevant facts.

In addition to the material written expressly for this book, I have included some of the papers or parts thereof that originally appeared in social science, medical, and plastic surgery journals or books. I have brought them together so that they will be accessible to a wider audience. This includes psychiatrists, mental health and social workers, nurses, teachers, and all those concerned with rehabilitation, as well as facially deviant persons and their families. Intended at the time for special and different audiences, these writings contained inevitable repetitions. To eliminate these and bring the articles into sharper focus for this book, deletions and revisions have been made, except in those instances where the trend of thought would be destroyed or the content altered.

For their support of much of my research I am indebted to the National Institute of Mental Health, United States Public Health Service, the Milbank Memorial Fund, The Association for the Aid of Crippled Children, and the Society for the Rehabilitation of the Facially Disfigured. The opportunity to work on this volume was made possible by a Special Fellowship Award from the Social Rehabilitation Service, United States Department of Health, Education, and Welfare.

My special appreciation goes to Dr. John Marquis Converse, Director of the Institute of Reconstructive Plastic Surgery, New

York University Medical Center, for our many years of association, and his cooperation and staunch support of my research since its inception. I am grateful to Mary E. Switzer, the late Commissioner of the United States Vocational Rehabilitation Administration, for her continued interest and her encouragement to do this book. To my teacher, colleague, and friend, Margaret Mead, I owe particular thanks. My early training under her auspices in addition to her special insights and wisdom have been of inestimable value. I owe much, too, to my former research assistant, Kathleen Kelly, for her unflagging assistance in checking masses of data and the details of earlier papers. For the laborious task of typing the manuscript I have to thank Janet Swords. I am greatly indebted to Helen MacGill Hughes for her editorial assistance on this particular volume. Her special expertise, enthusiasm, and encouragement have done much to lighten the task I have undertaken.

Finally, I am deeply grateful to the hundreds of patients and their families who have not only given me so much of their time, but, more important, for their confidence and willingness to discuss freely their feelings and experiences, painful as many of these were. From their collaboration it is our hope that others may benefit.

For permission to publish my papers as amended or adapted, I wish to acknowledge and thank the following: *The Journal of Health and Social Behavior, The American Sociological Review, The Angle Orthodontist, Plastic and Reconstructive Surgery, Psychosomatic Medicine*, W.B. Saunders Company, C.V. Mosby Company, The Russell Sage Foundation, and Williams and Wilkins Company.

Frances Cooke Macgregor
New York University Medical Center
Institute of Reconstructive
Plastic Surgery
New York City 1974

CHAPTER ONE

Face and Fate

THE CASE OF INGRID DE VALERY

> The face, in the final analysis, is the expression.
> The expression—how shall I put it—well, the
> expression is something like an equation by
> which we show our relationship with others.
> It's a roadway between oneself and others. If
> it's blocked by a landslide, even those who
> have been at pains to travel it will think you
> are now some uninhabited, delapidated house
> and perhaps pass by.
>
> (Kobo Abé, *The Face of Another*)

Ingrid was a wealthy and socially prominent woman of 33 who
came from France to New York for plastic surgery. Her face had
been terribly mutilated in an automobile accident thirteen years
before. She had undergone nineteen operations during the first two
years of her disfigurement, but, although these had accomplished
much in the way of jaw and dental reconstruction, her appearance was not markedly improved. In the following ten years she
had thirty more operations, but her face was still so marred that
she was called "la gueule cassée" (broken mug) in the city where
she lived.

The medical examination revealed that the middle portion of
Ingrid's face had been pushed backward causing a distortion of
its contour. The upper lip was carried upward and back, making
occlusion of the lips impossible. Because of the backward dis-
placement of the bones, two deep, unsightly folds marked each
side of the nose, which was shortened and twisted to one side. Her
left eye appeared to protrude and the lower lid to sag because of
the absence of bone support beneath the eye. She looked grotesque. Although her general health was good, she was susceptible
to anxiety states accompanied by palpitations and a feeling that
she lacked air. She did not sleep well, she smoked excessively, and
frequently indulged in periods of heavy drinking.

Had her face not been so misshapen, Ingrid's physical traits would have contributed greatly toward making her a handsome woman. She had exceptionally beautiful hair and a lithe, well-porportioned body. Furthermore, she enhanced her physical assets to their fullest extent by the meticulous care with which she dressed. Intelligent and prepossessing, she was obviously accustomed to dominating the situation, wherever she found herself. Her manner, charm, and grooming compelled attention and set her off as a person of distinction. She alternated between moods when she was irritable, tense, exacting, and vindictive and moods when she was vivacious, gay, and flirtatious.

Ingrid was anxious about her face. For twelve years she had lived under the strain of her unsightly appearance, yet she had striven desperately to overcome her handicap. But the mental strain was too great—"I am tired of always trying to be charming, to compensate for what I lack. It is such an endless effort. If only my face could be made to look normal enough for me to be able to sit back and rest once in a while and not always force myself to be entertaining or interesting and to create an atmosphere which will distract others from my disfigurement." She was prepared to "go through anything" that would help her appearance. She would stay in America for more than a year if necessary for the required operations, though it would mean being away from her two sons. Nor was the excessive cost of such work a deterrent. She demanded full and undivided attention from those in whose hands she placed herself. If she did not like someone called in for medical consultation or assistance, she found fault with him, complained, and demanded that another take his place.

Ingrid was born in Finland. She had one sister six years older than herself. Her father, a man of the upper class with considerable wealth, was well known in European business circles for his business acumen. A domineering person of strong convictions, he was intolerant of failure or weakness in himself or others. Her mother, according to Ingrid, was superficial, interested only in the social life that accompanied her elevated position.

As a small child Ingrid loved both her parents who, however, were in continual conflict with each other. This worried her. Frightened by the arguments that she heard from their rooms at night, she would get on her knees and pray that they would stop quarreling and be happy together. As she grew older, Ingrid favored her father. She still admires his strong character and his ability, although his occasional severity made her feel bitter toward him. For her mother, whom she described as a silly woman, Ingrid had little affection. Between Ingrid and her sister Karen, who was usually away at school, there was no real companionship. Ingrid does recall being shy with her because, when at home, Karen dominated her; she also remembers envying Karen's horsemanship and prize-winning ability at a time when Ingrid herself was too young to enter contests. Even at the time of this writing, she feels little affection for Karen.

Like most Finnish children, Ingrid was expected to be proficient in athletics. Her father, who taught her to swim in the coldest water almost as soon as she could walk, to throw the javelin, to ride, and to sail a boat, insisted that she master these skills, and he made no concession to pain or weakness. When she was 9 years old, her sister shoved the sailboat in which she was playing into the channel leading out to sea. Rather than let Karen know she was afraid, Ingrid sang as loudly as she could while the boat was carried swiftly away. Her father was forced to go to her rescue, yet nothing was made of the episode. "I was taught to play to win, to be a Spartan. To complain of a headache, to be frightened, to give up a contest was unthinkable."

Ingrid was adept in sports and happiest when playing with boys, because the "competition was keener." They would go into the nearby woods and play Indians. At that time stories about Indians and pioneering days in America were extremely popular with Ingrid and her friends. An especial devotee of Buffalo Bill, she always insisted upon taking his role. For years, she said, he was her ideal. Always wanting to be brave and Spartan-like, she felt that any display of interest in dolls was a sign of weakness. She hid hers in the closet, but secretly she loved them and brought them out when alone at night "for a few coveted moments."

Recounting how once her nurse had come upon her playing with her dolls, she said, "I was consumed with shame at having my weakness detected."

Ingrid joined the Girl Scouts and became head of her troop. At this period Scout activities were her greatest joy, for not only could she go camping, but "I could be like all the other girls, could wear a uniform, and do what they did without being followed around all the time by a governess."

Most of Ingrid's childhood was spent either moving with her parents from their city residence to their country estate, or going with them to various fashionable spas in Europe, following the social season. A French governess was in charge of her schooling. For a few months she attended a private school, but she did not like the teachers—"I hated to be dominated by them." Also, she was embarrassed by the expensive clothes in which her mother dressed her. She wanted to wear the simple frocks the other girls wore—"We had too much money and I didn't want the fact to be so evident to others."

When she was 13, her parents divorced and they placed her in a convent in Rome; however, her schooling was constantly interrupted at their whims. She was never in school for more than two consecutive months. One parent would suddenly send for her to come to Paris, or the other to Finland. "I was sent back and forth as one sends clothes—on approval." While at the convent, she often escaped and went to an artists' colony where she had a number of friends, for she preferred painting to study. She broke so many rules that she was finally dismissed. Sent to another convent, she continued to disobey rules. "As soon as I knew I could not do a thing, I wanted to do it." She disliked the nuns and the regimentation and within a few months was transferred to art school.

Ingrid was now 14, a gay, impetuous, and proficient sportswoman. She was also growing into a beautiful woman and was becoming aware of it—"I could see myself in the mirror." Men much older than she were beginning to be very attentive. Her mother, fearful that she would become too impressed by her attraction for men, endeavored to warn her by saying, "It is only because you're beautiful that they like you. If you were not, none of them would pay any attention to you." When a young man fell in love with her, her mother said, "He does not really love you; it is only your beauty he loves." Deciding to test this statement, Ingrid cut off all her hair and "the boy promptly lost interest."

At 17 she married a Swedish youth of her social class. She was happy with him and extremely pleased when her son was born a year later. Her happiness was short-lived, however, for she discovered that her husband was unfaithful to her. She decided to divorce him. Her father threatened to disown her for this, saying it was a foolish thing to do, but she did it anyway. Taking her baby and nurse with her, she went to live in the south of France. It was here two years later that she was in the accident that so seriously maimed her.

Ingrid had been seeing much of a young man who was intemperate in his affection for her and who had, on occasion, threatened to kill them both if she did not marry him. She had refused, although she continued to see him. On this day they had gone driving and no arguments had marred their afternoon together. Suddenly the car left the road. The young man was instantly killed. His mother still believes he crashed the car on purpose; Ingrid insists it was an accident.

For nearly two years, Ingrid was hospitalized. She had sustained multiple compound fractures of the facial bones. Both legs were severely fractured and for many months there was danger of her losing one. From the shock she was blind for almost a year, during which her face was enclosed in a cast up to her eyes. The physical and psychological trauma from which she suffered, the intense pain, and her inability to eat caused her weight to drop from 150 to 60 pounds. From the way her face felt, and the daily concern and attention given her by specialists brought in for consultation, she knew, though she could not see, that her face was "ruined." There were also the things she overheard: Discussing her condition, nurses used the term "ecrasé" (ruined). The extreme pity in the voices of her family and friends, and such remarks as "Poor Ingrid, how can you have the will to live?" left no doubt in her mind as to what had happened to her face. She felt, as she put it, "dead inside." As her sight slowly returned,

Ingrid studied her blurred image in the mirror every day. Her face was terribly swollen and her left eye protruded from its socket. Her lips no longer met, but hung apart revealing a pushed-in upper jaw and teeth that had turned yellow. Her nose was twisted upward and to one side. She could hold nothing between her lips and could open her jaws just enough to drink through a straw. For a year she had to spend time each day prying them apart—"I was terrible looking. I had a carnival face."

Concerning the future Ingrid decided she had three alternatives: "I could kill myself, I could enter a cloister where I would be hidden from the world and where I could work, or I could go back into the world and begin another life as an ugly woman." For several months she seriously considered the convent, for how could she go out into society again with such a face? During this critical period her family and friends tried to encourage her—"When you feel people love you, it gives value to life." In addition, a handsome young French aristocrat who had been in love with her before the accident visited her every day and begged her to marry him. "The fact that I was no longer beautiful seemed to make no difference to him. He never mentioned my face, he was kind, he waited on me constantly and I grew to love him." To marry him Ingrid had to become a Catholic. Never a very religious person, she says she now found "comfort and solace" in study and prayer. Under these various influences she gradually determined to make the best of things.

Fearful, however, that her friends might become "tired and bored" visiting her so often, she decided that her hospital room would be known for its gaiety. She tried to be humorous; she kept champagne on hand as a "kind of inducement" so they would know they could "always get a drink—and that helped."

On her release from the hospital Ingrid was married. The wealth and the social prominence that she and her husband commanded in European society obliged them to lead an active social life that she was determined to pursue—"Nothing would be avoided because of my face." There were receptions, evenings at the opera, and fashionable resorts they were expected to frequent. At first, she found social affairs extremely difficult:

I would look at myself in the mirror and think "How can I go out on the street with this awful face? What kind of clothes can I wear that will not make me look ridiculous? What kind of hat can be worn with a face like this?" I knew that now I must do everything possible to make myself presentable and to distract attention from my face. I must keep my hands and nails just so, wear the most beautiful but simple clothes, pay great attention to my hair, wear the most attractive perfumes—everything to help myself look interesting. But these things were not enough. Before my accident I had only been interested in having fun: occasional love affairs, traveling, and sports. I had few intellectual interests. Now I realized I must read everything new that came out, be well versed in the important topics of the time, be more gay and amusing than ever before. I must win people with my charm.

There was seldom a day when Ingrid did not go out, although "it was terribly hard to be stared at" everywhere she went. At the same time not to be recognized was a "devastating" experience. On one occasion she met an old friend who had not heard of her accident, and she was forced to tell him who she was. "He was so embarrassed (and so was I) that I decided I would never speak first to anyone again." Returning home to Finland for a visit, she found that other friends passed her on the streets without knowing who she was. Wherever she went she noticed people staring and talking among themselves about her. At a dinner party one evening she overheard a woman say, "How can she go out with a face like that?" Despite "feeling sick inside," she behaved as though she hadn't noticed. "I had to pretend to be gay at any price. I knew they were always thinking 'poor girl,' and I hate pity. It is most difficult to make people forget you are ugly and the only way you can is to show them you are happier now than ever before, that everything is easy and wonderful. People are jealous of others. If I could make them think 'she may be ugly but she is happier than anyone,' then they would envy me instead of pitying me."

When Ingrid was 23 she bore another son. A year later her homeland was at war. "Fanatically patriotic," she left her husband

and children and went to Finland where she drove an ambulance for four months. "I loved the danger of being in the midst of fighting." Soon afterward her husband, who had by now joined the French army, was wounded. For a year Ingrid nursed him, but during this time she began to lose respect for him. He constantly complained about his wounds and worried because he would have a slight limp. He became "entirely absorbed in himself." When the war economy cut off their income, he was indifferent to his family's plight. He joined the underground movement, and Ingrid took the children to Switzerland. Her ability to speak several languages, her business astuteness, and her wide acquaintance with influential people she had known through her father (no longer living) enabled her to develop rapidly a flourishing enterprise of trading on a commission basis. She also helped in the underground movement, frequently crossing the French border to carry out dangerous assignments.

During the critical war years Ingrid worried less about her face. "We never knew how long we would be alive. A pretty face was not so essential." But now the war was over, traveling and social activities would be resumed. Separated from her husband, she "had to make a lot of money." She wanted to live as fully as possible and she insisted that a presentable face was "imperative." She began her search for someone who could help her. Hearing of a highly recommended American surgeon, she flew to New York for a consultation.

The work on Ingrid's face was a slow and torturous process. Seventeen operations were performed, each requiring from two days to a week in the hospital. In addition, thirty-three anesthesias were administered for minor adjustments. She was never fearful of a pending operation, even though it might require many hours. "The pain and inconvenience is so insignificant compared to what may be gained. No one knows what it is like to go around looking like an old monkey, to feel as though you were diving into cold water every time you enter a room full of people."

When not hospitalized, Ingrid pursued her business activities. Driven by her desire to make money, at which she was highly successful, she spared herself no hardship. Once, though she was in pain from recent surgery on her nose, she flew to Europe for a week to take care of some important interests.

> I must have money in order to have power. With money one can do anything. Unless I can live well I refuse to live at all. If I were still beautiful, money would not be so important, but with a bad face and no money you are nothing. No one would help you, not even your closest friends. They cannot be counted upon as much as money. They will ask you to stay with them a week or a month, but that is not a lifetime, and you have to take care of yourself. One must be realistic and face facts. Life is not beautiful, but you can make it easier if you have money. I never want to be dependent upon anyone again.

She enjoyed being clever in business dealings. "I love the competition and I hate to be beaten at anything. I am like my father; I am hard and ruthless with those who are not my friends."

Ingrid had American acquaintances and as a person of influence and prominence received many invitations. At first she was reluctant to attend large parties or to dine in public. Her initial experiences in America made her feel that she was even more of a curiosity than she had been in Europe. People "seemed to stare" at her more, and they made remarks to her. In a drugstore a man had said, "We have hospitals and convalescent homes where people like you can go and where you can avoid being out in public." A waiter in a restaurant where she had been several times commented, "You are a great lady to go out in public with such a handicap. I could never do it." A woman clerk asked, "How are you able to make yourself go out with such a face?" Such incidents made Ingrid dread going anywhere. She walked along the streets in a slinking manner, keeping her head turned toward the shop windows to avoid being noticed. She grew more irritable and impatient and began to drink more than usual. But she refused to be defeated—"One can't give up. There is nothing else to do. You have to go on pretending you don't notice and never show you feel inferior." This refusal to be vanquished or to exhibit any weakness was a standard she did not confine to herself. She regarded weakness and lack of courage in others with equal contempt. Asked to talk with a war victim whose face had been as severely disfigured as her own and who was so depressed that he was threatening suicide, she ended her visit with him in disgust. "He only feels sorry for himself. All he wants to do is die or to hide somewhere because he is afraid others will feel sick at the sight of him. People have told me that the sight of my face made them sick. If that is the way they felt, I told them to leave me. I didn't want them around. You can't die. You must find a place for yourself."

Ingrid is what the French call "jolie laide"; those who meet her say that in a short time, by her charm, she can erase the features that at first sight are so repellent. This ability, deliberately cultivated, she used to the fullest extent. Ever since her disfigurement she has made a special effort to attract men—"I like to know I have power over them." A sexually sophisticated woman, she has been successful in gaining their attention. "My ability to do so makes other women jealous," she says. "And," she adds proudly, "one woman told me 'with your terrible face you can have all the men you want. I don't see how you do it.'" She enjoys telling of her "many conquests" of prominent men who wanted to be with her or marry her. She says she does not intend to marry again—"I never want to depend again on a man for money"—but she does enjoy occasional love affairs. She attributes her ability to attract men to her intelligence and charm—"Men like me because I am smart and gay. With a man you must have a sense of humor; you must never speak of your nose or your disfigurement. It would make him sick. You must make him forget your ugliness." Occasionally, however, she has felt utterly hopeless and inadequate, for the most unbearable part of being facially disfigured is, she says, "to have the man you love wake up to find such a face next to him."

Ingrid's desire to dominate was not limited to men who were sexually interested in her but included all others with whom she came in contact. She demanded and usually got what she wanted from them. Even in her relationships with women she insisted on being in control. Particularly attracted to goodlooking women, she made as much effort to charm them as she did men. Admiring their physical beauty and fearing it at the same time, she became angry if they did not accede to her impulsive wishes or if they showed what she considered "too much independence." In all personal relationships she was quick to see and to point out defects in others. These defects she discussed freely with persons she knew had high regard for the one under discussion. Not only did she focus attention upon their imperfections, but often distorted information in order to create dissension.

As the months passed, Ingrid's face began to show remarkable improvement. Her lips were brought together and the protrusion of her eye was corrected. To give her nose a normal contour an acrylic support, which could be inserted into the nasal cavity, was attached to the upper denture, an extremely difficult, not to mention humiliating, type of prosthesis for her to remove and reinsert daily. Ingrid was, nevertheless, pleased with the cosmetic effect. Although her reflection in the mirror gave irrefutable evidence of the changes taking place, she craved favorable comment from others. Even exaggerated flattery, which she recognized as such, was welcome. If improvement was not immediately noticed and remarked upon, she became angry and depressed.

At the end of a year Ingrid's face had been so transformed that with the exception of her nose, which was still noticeably damaged, she was no longer "la gueule cassée," but a presentable woman. With her nose covered by a small bandage, a device she had never before used because "there was too much to cover," the rest of her features appeared to be relatively normal. At discharge the surgeon told her that the prognosis for further improvement was not favorable. She felt that if nothing more could ever be done, she would resign herself to that fact and continue to live as fully as possible: "What else can you do? Life is too short and one must make the most of it. With such a face as I have had, one learns to have the courage to play the loser."

Twenty-four Years Later

Today Ingrid is a grandmother. In the intervening years she has had several minor operations; while she has long since discarded the covering on her nose, it remains noticeably foreshortened and she still needs to wear her cumbersome prosthesis. Nevertheless, Ingrid has managed, outwardly at least, to maintain her spirit and zest for excitement.

Her estrangement from her husband led to a divorce. Then as if to keep from dwelling on her face, she began to travel widely, if capriciously, about the world, visiting friends and acquaintances at fashionable watering places, and seeking adventure. There were times, too, when her drinking seemed to be on the increase causing concern among her friends. Meanwhile her style and confident manner continued to intrigue men and she eventually remarried, this time to a wealthy Englishman. Now married about fifteen years, Ingrid is still restless and independent; despite her husband and home, she views herself as "the eternal vaga-bond." But behind her seeming gaiety and lack of self-pity —"with my strange face I am not doing too badly"—is the never relinquished hope for further improvement.

THE CASE OF MARY AMRYSH

> When in disgrace with fortune and men's eyes,
> I all alone beweep my outcast state.
>
> (Shakespeare, SONNET XXIX)

Forty-three-year-old Mary Amrysh was born with a facial anomaly known as ocular hypertelorism.[1] In addition to this affliction she had a cleft lip and bilateral cleft of the nose. By comparison with photographs taken when she was 10 years old, her appearance had been markedly altered by a series of fifteen surgical procedures performed over several years. The gaping hole in the middle of her face had been closed, but, with respect to the total configuration, the improvements were only relative. She still presented a startling and gargoyle-like appearance. Her small, abnormally shaped eyes were set far to each side of her broad

---

[1] A craniofacial deformity characterized by defective development of the sphenoid bone and great breadth of the bridge of the nose with correspondingly great width between the eyes; it is a congenital condition.

face. Her nose, which lacked a bridge, was a formless mass and her mouth was off center. A noticeable growth of hair on her upper lip added to her unsightly appearance. She was a strong-looking, heavy, large-boned woman and, though poorly dressed, took care to appear clean and neat. Although her education had been meagre, she was fairly intelligent and responsive.

At her initial interview, Mary was tearful and distraught. Because of her face she had been denied throughout her entire life the opportunity to live as others do and was forced to endure the endless humiliation and indignity of being regarded as a freak. She declared she had reached the "breaking point"—"I feel so badly," she said. "Wherever I go I feel so out of place."

She had come to the plastic surgery clinic hoping that something could be done to make her more acceptable. All she asked for was to be improved enough so she could obtain a self-supporting job. "I'd like to get one in a factory and work like other people, support myself decently and better myself. I just make enough working in a laundry to pay my room rent and meals. I can't buy any clothes or save any money for my old age. I'm geting older and no one will want to take care of me." Whenever she tried to get a better job she was turned down. "And yet," she stated, "I am strong, I have hands, and I can work." Though eligible for state aid she had rejected help as well as a suggestion to go to a Catholic agency—"I'd rather starve or die on the street than ask them for anything. I want to take care of myself."

Mary was the eldest of four children. Her Czechoslovakian-born parents were poor and uneducated. The family lived in a poor section on the outskirts of a large city. Her father, who worked in a lumbermill, died when she was 10. "He should have done something for me when I was young. But he was too stupid; he didn't know any better. My mother said he always objected to the idea of my having any operations." Although the eldest child, Mary slept with her mother—"I always wanted to be with her. I never got along with my two brothers or my sister because I didn't see why I had to look the way I did or why I couldn't be like them."

She remembers that in her early childhood her mother kept her in the backyard because other people called her "funny." For four years Mary went to a parochial school but was withdrawn for reasons she claims not to know, although one feels fairly sure it was because of matters related to her affliction. When her mother tried to enroll her in a public school, the teacher insisted that Mary first have her harelip corrected because they "were afraid that other children would make fun of me." Although Mrs. Amrysh was resistant to the suggestion—"she was an uneducated woman and thought the doctors would practice on me"—Mary was taken to the city hospital. A year later, when she was 11, Mary entered public school—"But the children made fun of me because I was bigger and older than they were."[2]

Meanwhile Mrs. Amrysh was working in a carpet factory to support her family, and Mary took care of the younger children. "I stayed home from school a lot, maybe because of the other children; they made fun of me. I never liked school; I never liked anything; I never liked myself." Held back by frequent hospitalizations and her voluntary absences from school, Mary didn't graduate from the grammar grades until she was 16. During these years, instead of playing with others after school, she went home and remained indoors. But she remembers warmly the two "friends" she did have. In the fourth grade she became so attached to the Sister who was "nice" to her that she refused advancement to the next grade. She also recalled with deep affection a public school teacher who had been good to her—"She used to take me to her home and teach me how to knit. She was kind to me. She went to China thirty years ago and I still write to her. Anyone who is nice to me I get attached to. If they're mean, I never forget."

Once Mary and her sister were invited to visit an aunt; her sister refused to take Mary, who cried and said, "I know it's because I'm not good enough to go with you." "I never forgave her, and I really hated her because she was pretty and I wasn't.

---

[2] It is not uncommon for severely disfigured persons who are struggling to preserve their self-esteem to skirt (outside a clinical context) direct reference to the face and to attribute their difficulties to other characteristics. For example, a girl with a gross facial anomaly and malformed but functionally normal hands never once indicated that her grave social problems were related to her horrendous facial appearance. Only after marked surgical improvements were made could she speak of her face.

When my mother asked me to do anything for her I'd say, 'Let Alice do it, she's more beautiful than I am.' Even today, the minute I see her, I can't stand the sight of her."

Mary said she often reproached her mother about her deformity and told her she would be better off dead—"You should have stopped feeding me; it would have been better than going through life like this." On such occasions Mrs. Amrysh would cry, or say, "Someday you will have children and you'll understand how I feel."

Mary did not want to go to high school; she wanted only to work and earn money to help her mother. But wherever she went people stared at her—"Children would stop playing and say to each other, 'Look at that woman with the funny face.' People often asked me what happened." Her answers, Mary said, depended upon her mood. "Sometimes I get so mad I say 'Mind your own business,' or I say 'I've been run over by a car,' or sometimes I tell the truth."

Mary wanted to work in the carpet factory where her mother worked and where there were some girls she knew. But she was told she "might get a cancer of the face from infection from the wool." At another factory, the examining physician gave her no reason for his refusal to pass her, though she was physically fit. She sought employment in laundries, but was turned down as an insurance risk—"They made plenty of excuses just to get rid of me." Sometimes she made her mother go with her while she sought employment. "I told her, 'You're so smart, you brought me into this world. Now you see it isn't easy for me to get a job.'" When her mother cried, Mary "felt bad" because she had blamed her.

She eventually secured a job in a hospital laundry but at a salary less than other girls performing the same duties. When she protested she was told that she was "lucky to get a job at all." Here she worked for five years and at another laundry for fifteen years, where she earned a minimum wage. Often the staring and questions of those about her and "the feeling that the other girls didn't want to work with me" became more than she could endure and she would quit in despair. But the realization that other jobs were unattainable drove her back to the laundry. Once she went to an agency to seek work as a housemaid. She was sent to a woman who "took one look at me and shut the door." At the agency Mary was told not to come back as they could not help her.

When Mary was 23 she underwent three more surgical procedures hoping that some improvement would result in a better chance of securing employment. Slight corrections were made, but not enough to make her more presentable. When she was 26 her mother died, and Mary had no more surgery—"I figured I had nothing to live for anymore. I didn't care if I worked or not. She was the only one who was good to me or took care of me. Once I lost her, I lost faith in everything and many times I thought of suicide." Meanwhile, Mary's sister, six years her junior, had had two sons born out of wedlock. Since Mary could not support herself adequately, it was decided that she would take care of the children (1 and 5 years old) while her sister went to work. For eight years Mary cared for the boys, becoming so attached to them that she felt as though they were her own.

When her sister married, her husband agreed to let Mary remain with them because "he didn't want people to think he had thrown me out." According to Mary, he "drank a lot and said mean things" to her, and there were constant arguments over the boys, whom he mistreated. "The oldest one goes to school and comes home crying because the other kids make fun of him. He makes faces when he talks so he can't go shopping and ask for things."

On her own initiative, she took the boy to a psychiatrist—"I didn't want him to suffer the way I have." When his parents discovered this they vigorously objected, saying the boy was not "crazy." When Mary reproached the step-father for calling the boys "stupid," more arguments ensued. One night he told her, "A person with a face like yours should be destroyed," and ordered her to leave the house. "He is just an ignorant 'Polack,'" Mary said, but she wept at the thought of being kept away from the boys. "It was," she said, "the last straw. They were all I had—when I took them to the park, if other children made remarks about my face they always said, 'Don't mind them.'"

Mary moved to a small room and got a job in the laundry of a home for the blind. "I feel better when I see blind people because they are worse off than I am."

Mary says she has a couple of girl friends who work in the carpet factory who are nice to her—"They say they don't understand why I can't get a job in their factory. They say, 'You have two eyes, two hands, you can talk and think, why shouldn't you be able to work there?'" Sometimes they invite her to their homes, but she feels that when they go out, they don't want her around. Occasionally they go to a movie, but she dislikes eating in public places afterward. "People stare and I feel they don't want to eat after me; they probably think I have a disease. I guess I'd feel the same way, though." Mary is only too well aware of her repelling face and takes pains to avoid her own reflected image. "I can't remember when I last looked in a mirror. I never use one to comb my hair, and I can shave the hair on my upper lip without one. I don't care how I look. I can't buy clothes anyway—I have no money. I just try to keep myself neat and clean."

Following her examination at the plastic surgery clinic, it was decided that, because of the amount of scar tissue from earlier operations, no further surgery should be attempted.

At what was to be our last interview Mary was depressed and angry and felt that "life is not worth living. I can't go out in the world and I can't get work." Just traveling on the train to the clinic was, because of the staring, an "ordeal" she could no longer tolerate. "I used to talk with my priest for comfort. He once sent me to a woman who needed a helper in her home. When she saw me she said, 'I have two children and I can't hire you.' When I tell my priest my troubles he says I imagine things. He hasn't been around; he doesn't know what I go through. It makes me so mad when he tells me that. I don't go to church any more. I've given up hope." Breaking into tears she said, "I always wish the Lord would take me. He took my mother and father, and left me in this world by myself." It was quite clear that she meant what she said. When she read in the papers that a woman was convicted for having killed her deformed child, she wrote a letter to the judge. "I sent him my picture. I asked him what such a child could have to live for and said that I wished that woman had been my mother."

At the termination of the interview Mary was taken by the clinic's sociologist to see Henry Viscardi at the Institute of Physical Medicine and Rehabilitation. Mr. Viscardi was at the time the Executive Director of JOB (Just One Break), a newly organized program designed to help the physically handicapped to find employment, for, although not physically disabled, Mary was undoubtedly disabled occupationally.

Mr. Viscardi's concern with the occupational plight of the handicapped was intense and highly personal.[3] Born with dwarfed misshapen legs he had spent his first twenty-five years viewing the world from his diminished (3½-foot) body, with all that this entails. Eventually fitted with prosthetic legs he now gave the impression of a physically normal man.

Mary wept briefly while telling him her troubles. Tears came also to Mr. Viscardi's eyes when she described some of her experiences. "You know," he said, "I'm beginning to think that the problems of those with cosmetic defects are in some ways more serious than those of other physically handicapped people." He was frank in telling Mary that he did not know how he could help her but hoped in time that the public could be educated enough to make life less difficult for those with facial deviations. He did suggest, however, that she let him know if she should hear of an opening in the carpet factory where she wanted to work, in which case he would contact the head of the company. Mary seemed extremely pleased by his kindness and remarked that at the last employment agency visited "the man in charge wouldn't sit and talk to me the way you're doing." Mr. Viscardi replied, "Looking at you does not disturb me. I know that underneath you have the same heart and mind that I do."

As Mary entered the elevator with the sociologist on leaving, a striking example of the involuntary, visceral reaction of many

[3] See Viscardi, Jr., Henry, *A Man's Stature*. John Day Company, New York, 1952.

people to an unsightly face occurred. No remarks were made, nothing was said, but a woman passenger upon seeing Mary went white and turned her whole body toward the wall. This act took place in the matter of seconds but did not go unobserved. Mary looked at the sociologist with an expressionless face, but in that second her eyes seemed to say, "You see, this is what I go through all the time."

CHAPTER TWO

Appearance,
Interaction,
and Identity

THE SOCIAL SIGNIFICANCE OF THE FACE

> The recognition of the role of visibility in social perception makes possible the explanation of very important aspects in the dynamics of human relations.
> (Gustav Ichheiser, *Misunderstandings in Human Relations. A Study in False Social Perception*, American Journal of Sociology.)

As the two preceding histories demonstrate, we live in a world in which the way we look makes a difference in the responses we get. In an investigation of the problems of the facially disfigured, therefore, it is not enough to inquire into matters of social participation, acceptance and rejection, personality adjustment, and other concomitant phenomena. One must also ask the fundamental question: Why is the human face of such profound social significance? What is there about a facial deformity that makes it one of the most devastating of social handicaps?

That other types of physical deviations may become handicaps is easily understood. In the blind, the fact of blindness makes unnecessary any explanation of his handicap: It is apparent that the act of seeing is indispensable to the carrying out of the ordinary activities of daily life. The one-armed person or someone crippled by arthritis or cardiac disease is incapacitated to a greater or less degree also, and many of his activities are circumscribed because of his physical state. The social significance of these disabilities is obvious. On the other hand, a person with a facial disfigurement that affects normal expressive movements or mars the appearance does not necessarily suffer from any sensory defect, nor from any functional impairment that would ipso facto prevent his participation in the same pursuits as other people. Nevertheless, he is generally considered socially unacceptable, or made to feel so, and is classified as handicapped.

Why this should be so seems obvious: The man's face is repellent. It is ugly. His expression is distorted. He is not "good to look at." In other words, he becomes handicapped because of his appearance rather than because of a functional or organic impairment, which other types of physically handicapped people have in common. The issue therefore seems to be one of esthetic values. Yet this is not a complete explanation. The question still remains: Of what social significance is the face that damage to it should generally be of greater consequence than, for example, an ugly disfigurement of the same degree in another part of the body?

INTERPRETATIONS OF THE FACE

The human face is a complexity of far-reaching meaningfulness. As a visible clue to the "inner life" and a significant social stimulus, it has intrigued men throughout recorded history and played a crucial role in human behavior. From its contour, features, and expressions, conclusions are drawn about character, emotions, intellectual endowments, and cultural background. As far back as written records go, and even in ancient folklore,[1] references are found that appraise or interpret the face of a man as an indicator of the man himself. So significant are facial structure, features, and expressions that they have interested men not only in face-to-face encounters and interchange, but also as objects of serious study from many different perspectives and for many different purposes.

Physiognomy, the art of discovering characteristics of the personality from outward appearance with special attention to the configuration and expression of the face, has probably always been practiced.[2] In this connection, one of the earliest objective studies of the face was made by Aristotle, whose somewhat fanci-

[1] Burr, Charles W., "Personality and Physiognomy," in *The Human Face: A Symposium*. The Dental Cosmos, Philadelphia, 1935, p. 81.

[2] Allport, Gordon W., *Personality: A Psychological Interpretation*. Henry Holt and Company, New York, 1937, p. 65.

ful observations and character assessments are not markedly different from those we hear today.[3] He concluded:

Men with small foreheads are fickle, whereas if they are rounded or bulging out, the owners are quick tempered. Straight eyebrows indicate softness of disposition, those that curve out toward the temples, humor and dissimulation. The staring eye indicates impudence, the winking, indecision. Large and outstanding ears indicate a tendency to irrelevant talk and chattering.[4]

On the subject of noses, he was even more specific. Insensitive and swinish persons had, he claimed, thick, bulbous noses; the irascible, sharp-tipped noses; the magnanimous, rounded and large noses; and those of luxurious habits had snub noses. Open nostrils were a sign of passion.

Elsewhere in the Greek classics are allusions to the practice of physiognomy and to the determination of character by outward appearance. Cleanthes, the Stoic, maintained that it was possible to tell a person's habits from the aspect of his face, and Socrates was supposed to have recognized the abilities of Plato at first glance.

During the Aristotelian revival in the thirteenth century, the treatise *Physiognomonica*, attributed to Aristotle, which contained a list of sources from which physiognomic signs were drawn,[5] precipitated not only a renewed interest in physiognomy but served as a stimulus for fraudulent occupations that have flourished ever since. Quacks and charlatans, quick to see the rich possibilities in divination and character reading, became such a menace that by 1743, during the reign of George II, it became a punishable offense for anyone to pretend to be skilled in it. Encouraged by a credulous and unenlightened public, however, the dubious trade continues into the present day.

But there were others who had more serious and scientific pur-

[3] Such beliefs are not confined to the superstitious or uneducated. During this investigation a scholar was heard to remark, "Men whose heads are flat in the back cannot be trusted."

[4] Aristotle, "Historia Animalium" Oxford Translation of 1910, cited by Charles W. Burr, loc. cit.

Macalister, Alexander, "Physiognomy," *Encyclopaedia Britannica*, eleventh edition, vol. 21, 1911, pp. 550–552.

[5] Allport, Gordon W., op. cit., p. 66.

poses in view. In 1772 Johann Casper Lavater, founder of the so-called science of physiognomy, produced his *Physiognomical Bible*. In this work, he ascribed to man special "physiognomical sensations" that consisted of "those feelings which are reproduced at beholding certain countenances, and the conjectures conveying the qualities of the mind, which are produced by the state of such countenances, or of their portraits drawn or painted."[6]

The study of expressions of the face (which is said to be capable of 250,000 different expressions)[7] first achieved a truly scientific foundation in 1806 when Charles Bell, an English surgeon, wrote *The Anatomy and Philosophy of Expression*. This was followed in 1872 by Darwin's well-known study, *The Expression of the Emotions in Man and Animals*, which stimulated interest and research particularly among psychologists. Thus physiognomy, for all its checkered and somewhat shadowy history, has nevertheless become an important branch of the psychology of personality. Despite the unfounded and naive observations of earlier writers, many of whose notions still enjoy wide acceptance, it is "a challenging fact that men have always found some indirect assistance in their judgements of others through the observation of their physical expressions: their eyes, their cast of countenance, their facial play, their posture, build and manner. . . . The face seems to betray one's way of life."[8]

Among others who have attempted to learn about man from his face are the anthropologists, who have concerned themselves with proportions, nasal contour, skin texture, color, and so on, of racial types. Lombroso, the Italian criminologist, whose ideas are now largely superseded, attempted to prove that criminals belong to a distinct anthropological type with distinctive and inherited craniofacial stigmata. Psychiatrists, stimulated by Kretschmer's theory of the relation between the face and affective personalities, have

---

[6] Lavater, Johann Casper, *Physiognomical Bible* (1772), cited by Leo Kanner, "Judging Emotions from Facial Expression," in *Psychological Monographs*, No. 41, Psychological Review Company, Princeton, New Jersey, 1931, p. 2.

[7] Birdwhistell, Ray L., *Kinesics and Context: Essays on Body Motion Communication*. University of Pennsylvania Press, Philadelphia, 1970, p. 8.

[8] Allport, Gordon W., op. cit., p. 67.

turned their attention to it as an indicator of mental illness, and have sought in facial deviations the genesis of psychoses.[9] Anatomists[10] and paleontologists[11] have considered it in its anatomical and phylogenic aspects, physicians with reference to possible diagnostic clues,[12] and plastic surgeons from the viewpoint of repair and reconstruction.[13]

Interest in the human face has not been confined to scientists and pseudo-scientists, as any brief survey of literature and art will confirm. For centuries it had been a primary subject of interest in sculpture and painting, and studied minutely. The infinite variety of its contours and expressions has provided an inexhaustible source of material to artists whose aims range from merely getting a likeness to capturing the essential personality of the model. Nor has the face been neglected in literature. Poets have glorified its beauty and have tried to capture through the medium of words the ethical qualities, temperament, or personality as revealed by the face and its expressive features[14]:

> And on that cheek and o'er that brow,
> So soft, so calm, yet eloquent,
> The smiles that win, the tints that glow
> But tell of days in goodness spent,
> A mind at peace with all below,
> A heart whose love is innocent.
>   —Lord Byron

[9] Updegraff, Howard L., and Karl A. Menninger, "Some Psychoanalytic Aspects of Plastic Surgery," *American Journal of Surgery*, vol. 25, September 1934, pp. 554–558.

[10] Huber, Ernst, *Evolution of Facial Musculature and Facial Expression*. The Johns Hopkins Press, Baltimore, 1931.

[11] Gregory, William K., *Our Face from Fish to Man*. G. P. Putnam's Sons, New York, 1929.

[12] Thorek, Max, *The Face in Health and Disease*. F. A. Davis and Company, Philadelphia, 1946.

[13] Kazanjian, Varaztad H., and John Marquis Converse, *The Surgical Treatment of Facial Injuries*, third edition. Williams & Wilkins Company, Baltimore, in press.

[14] Cooley noted that in *Familiar Quotations* "only four words, 'heart,' 'love,' 'man,' and 'world' were quoted more frequently than the word 'eye.'" Cooley, Charles H., *Human Nature and the Social Order*. Schocken New York, 1964, p. 108.

In such familiar and trite expressions as "the face is the mirror of the soul," "your face is your fortune," and "his face is an open book," social significance is exemplified, becoming even more meaningful when the face happens to be a misfortune.

By dictionary definition, a deformity is that which is misshapen, disfigured, which conspicuously departs from regularity, or deviates from what is deemed acceptable or beautiful. For this study, however, and for purposes of further delineation, facial deformity is defined as any physical deviation that differentiates the victim from others to the extent that it may be regarded as socially or psychologically handicapping. Exceedingly difficult if not impossible to conceal, deformities of the face have profound consequences for social identity and interaction. In this respect they do more damage than do defects of the same degree in other parts of the body and are the most common disfigurements that give rise to psychic distress. They may be socially handicapping, in some instances, to an even greater degree than a more radical defect in some other part of the body.

The individual with a facial deformity may be the object of ridicule or deprecatory jokes.[15] Or, since many people judge intelligence[16] and character by the face, the unfortunate possessor of a receding chin, lop ears, a paralyzed mouth, or crossed eyes may be thought of as stupid, insensitive, or even vicious. In addition, prejudice against facial stigmata based on the belief that they are caused by a disease, or by some "sin" committed by the possessor or his progenitors, is still prevalent. Some visual stimuli are responded to quite unconsciously, yet they subtly determine the

[15] In a classification of jokes about physically defective people, Barker, Wright, Meyerson, and Gonick found that 80 percent were of a deprecatory nature, and that 40 percent concerned facial defects. Barker, Roger G., Beatrice A. Wright, Lee Meyerson, and Mollie R. Gonick, *Adjustment to Physical Handicap and Illness: Social Psychology of Physique and Disability*. Social Science Research Council, Bulletin 55, New York, 1953, pp. 75–76.

[16] S. W. Cook found that those with symmetrical features and a pleasant expression were judged to be the highest in intelligence, while those judged low in intelligence had fat, oval, narrow, or lopsided faces, crossed eyes, larger noses, larger ears, thick lips, overhanging eyebrows, sunken eyes, or abnormally high eyebrows. Cook, Stuart W., "Judgment of Intelligence from Photographs," *Journal of Abnormal and Social Psychology*, vol. 34, no. 3, 1939, pp. 384–389.

impulse to approach or avoid the afflicted.[17] Aware that others are prone to judge him by his face and what his appearance signifies, the disfigured individual often feels incapable of revealing his real personality. Having no control over the way he looks he may be destined, like Victor Hugo's *L'Homme Qui Rit*, to a life fraught with misunderstanding.

THE FACE AND VISUAL IMPRESSION

A most important aspect of the social significance of the face is its role as a stimulus to visual impression. It is through the medium of the senses that men perceive their fellows. Also through the senses impressions are received that elicit affective responses of attraction and repulsion. From a person's face, the sound of his voice, and the touch of his hand, sense impressions are conveyed that produce emotional and esthetic attitudes in the beholder. But of all sense relationships affecting the intensity of social nearness or social distance between individuals, visual impressions predominate.[18] In this connection, the face as a social stimulus becomes of primary importance.

Because the face is intimately connected with communication, both verbal and nonverbal, and the region where the sense of selfhood is generally located,[19] it is for most people the center of attention in face-to-face interaction.[20] Moreover, it is a principal medium of emotional expression. As a receptor of impressions as well as a medium by which rejection, threat, or invitation may be

[17] Allport, Floyd H., *Social Psychology*. Johnson Reprint Corp., New York, 1967, p. 220.

[18] Park, Robert E., and Ernest W. Burgess, *Introduction to the Science of Sociology*. University of Chicago Press, Chicago, 1924, 1969, pp. 356–360; also Heritage of Sociology Series, University of Chicago Press.

[19] Allport, Gordon W., op. cit., p. 481.

[20] There are exceptions: for example, Taureg men of West Africa wear over their faces veils that conceal all but the area around the eyes. Identification is made from such clues as dress style, stature, hands, and feet. By making themselves faceless the Taureg are able to maintain social distance and a much coveted sense of privacy. Murphy, Robert F., "Social Distance and the Veil," *American Anthropologist*, vol. 66, no. 6, part I, 1964, pp. 1257–1274.

expressed, it is a dominant aspect in the interaction of individuals, serving to qualify the interplay between them and to influence communication. Together with the voice and body gestures, the face provides clues to the person himself. It becomes, in effect, a personal symbol by which one is able to bridge the gap between one mind and another. From the initial glance, the countenance becomes a vehicle for personal impressions and inferences, a basis of antipathy or sympathy, and a precipitant of a train of thought to better knowledge of the other. This perception of a person's individuality, which the face especially discloses, depends upon the eyes. Of the special sense organs, the eye, according to Simmel, has a unique sociological function:

The union and interaction of individuals is based upon mutual glances. This is perhaps the most direct and purest reciprocity which exists anywhere. . . . So tenacious and subtle is this union that it can only be maintained by the shortest and straightest line between the eyes, and the smallest deviation from it, the slightest glance aside, completely destroys the character of this union. . . . The interaction of eye to eye dies the moment in which the directness of the function is lost. But the totality of social relations of human beings, their self-assertion and self-abnegation, their intimacies and estrangements, would be changed in unpredictable ways if there occurred no glance of eye to eye.

By the glance which reveals the other, one discloses himself. By the same act in which the observer seeks to know the observed, he surrenders himself to be understood by the observer. The eye cannot take unless at the same time it gives. . . .

Shame causes a person to look at the ground to avoid the glance of the other. The reason for this is certainly not only because he is thus spared the visible evidence of the way in which the other regards his painful situation, but the deeper reason is that the lowering of his glance to a certain degree prevents the other from comprehending the extent of his confusion. The glance in the eye of the other serves not only for me to know the other but also enables him to know me. Upon the line which unites the two eyes, it conveys to the other the real personality, the real attitude, and the real impulse.[21]

[21] Simmel, Georg, *Soziologie.* Duncker und Humblot, Leipzig, 1908, pp. 646–651; cited in Park and Burgess, op. cit., pp. 358–59.
Among the Balinese, courtship is a matter of glances. The highest point is in the first glance, after which romantic excitement steadily dies down. Bateson, Gregory, and Margaret Mead, *Balinese Character.* New York Academy of Sciences, New York, 1942, p. 37.

The significance of the face as a source of impression formation and in influencing personal relationships becomes clear. Almost everyone coming in contact with a total stranger has experienced immediate feelings of like or dislike. How often have we heard it said of someone after a brief encounter, "There is something about him I don't like"? Such affective attitudes may evade description, yet are somehow linked with the "way he looks." By the briefest visual perception, a mental picture is formed of the kind of person he is. The first contact affords little opportunity to penetrate the personality deeply, or to discover contradictions of the first judgments: Subsequent interchanges and observation may confirm or alter these judgments, but unless the contact is resumed, the initial impression, right or wrong, is likely to remain.

The rapidity with which first impressions are formed, and the impulsive rather than critical judgments often made, operate to the disadvantage of those with facial defects. Since antipathies are related to the primary sense areas and are apparently devoid of reason, they may serve as barriers to the development of sympathetic social interaction.[22] The individual with an unattractive physical trait, therefore, may be the object of an immediate negative reaction even though it may be followed by realization that sympathy should have been awakened.[23] Whereas a marred face may not be so unsightly as to generate a visceral response, it may, nevertheless, serve as a misleading mask, which, despite efforts to render impartial and rational judgment, blinds others not only to the play of subtle and meaningful expressions, but to the real self behind the mask. Thus Allport speaks of "the undue constraint found frequently in perceptual processes, whereby some item in the field claims the observer's attention, and contributes disproportionately to the meaning aroused, quite eclipsing the evidence from the surrounding cues."[24]

---

[22] Alexander, Chester, "Antipathy and Social Behavior," *American Journal of Sociology*, vol. 51, no. 4, 1946, pp. 289–291.

[23] A facially disfigured war veteran reported the following incident: He had entered a bar and was standing at the counter to order a drink. The waitress whose back was turned at the time, upon seeing him gasped and put her hands to her face. A few minutes later she exclaimed, "Oh, that poor boy!"

[24] Allport, Gordon W., op. cit., p. 484.

The cues become what Allport terms "anchorage points," and from them no judgment is allowed to drift. Victim of just such misjudgment was Cyrano de Bergerac, whose immense and ugly nose gave no hint of the poetic soul underneath. Sensitive to the reactions his nose evoked and fearful of ridicule, he was impelled to express his deep feelings for the woman he loved through the mouth of a handsome man from whom words of endearment would seem more congruous.

Here, then, is the predicament of the facially disfigured. Usually unable to hide his defect, wearing it where all may see, his face is a visual stimulus to impressions and affective attitudes he is helpless to prevent. How he will react and adjust will depend both on himself and on the attitudes and behavior of others toward him.

CULTURAL CONCEPTS OF BEAUTY

Relevant to the social significance of the face is the concept of beauty. Beauty is a social phenomenon, and its importance in human life, as well as that of its counterpart, ugliness, cannot be underrated. As far as social stimuli are concerned, probably greater differentiation is made in human society between the physically attractive and the unattractive people than is drawn between the sexes.[25] Beauty can be, according to Schilder, a promise of complete satisfaction.

> Our own beauty or ugliness will not only figure in the image we get about ourselves but will also figure in the image others build up about us and which will be taken back into ourselves. The body image is the result of social life. Beauty and ugliness are certainly not phenomena in the single individual but are social phenomena of the utmost importance.[26]

[25] Perrin, F. A. C., "Physical Attractiveness and Repulsiveness," *Journal of Experimental Psychology*, vol. 4, June 1921, pp. 203–217.

[26] Schilder, Paul, *The Image and Appearance of the Human Body*. Psychological Monographs, No. 4, K. Paul, Trench, Trubner and Company, London, 1935, p. 267.

Physical characteristics exert a profound influence over one's associates. The fact that physically attractive people elicit favorable responses is obvious to anyone who has observed his fellow men. Physical qualities pleasing to see or to touch are definitely assets, not just in making their possessors more popular and more in demand than the physically repellent, with respect to sexual selection, but also in connection with those often overlooked but sociologically significant "small" phenomena of social life.[27] Since physical appeal is dependent in such large measure upon the face, particularly in societies where people are fully clothed, it has probably been given more attention than any other part of the body. A handsome person, regardless of what he may say or do, tends to evoke responses that are not what they would be were he ugly.

The esthetic interest in man's physical qualities is intimately connected with interest in sex, and consequently with an urgent human need. In most societies there is preference for a particular physical type, and in those that permit free choice of mates the preference plays an important role in social selection. Even in primitive communities, a handsome man, though he may not meet the requirements of a desirable husband, has a better chance than an ugly one to perpetuate his type. And in general, as in our society, the prettiest girls are sought by the ablest or wealthiest men, while the ugly ones must be content with inferiors.[28]

These culturally determined preferences for particular physical characteristics sometimes assume exceedingly vigorous forms. Among the Tanala of Madagascar, for example, were two groups of people whose physical characteristics were similar except for skin color: one group had light brown skin, the other dark brown. If a child of one shade of brown was born into a group of the other shade, though his parentage be unquestioned, he was put to

[27] Ichheiser, Gustav, "The Significance of the Physical Beauty of the Individual in Socio-Psychological and Sociological Explanation," *Zeitschrift für Völkerpsychologie und Soziologie*, September 1928, translated by E. C. Hughes in *An Introduction to Sociology*, revised edition, by Carl A. Dawson and Warner E. Gettys. The Ronald Press Company, New York, 1935, p. 751.

[28] Linton, Ralph, *The Study of Man*. Appleton-Century-Crofts, New York, 1936, 1964, p. 31.

death in the belief that if allowed to live he would become either a sorcerer, a leper, or a thief, or would be guilty of incest.[29] This form of social selection naturally affects the physical type of the group and is, as Linton suggests, one of the possible causes of man's present physical diversity.[30] Such "docility" of sex attraction has been used to explain the peculiar facial characteristics of the Basques, Armenians, and Jews, for, as isolated populations, they select mates according to their own accepted standards of beauty.[31]

Although beauty is so significant in human society, it is nevertheless very difficult to define. Not only do we lack specific measures of it, but we find that the concepts of that which is beautiful or even acceptable and that which is ugly or deviant are relative. Samuel Johnson contended that if we were more accustomed to deformity than beauty, the ideas now annexed to deformity would be attached to beauty. It is only because we are more accustomed to beauty that we approve it and admire it. "If a man, born blind, was to recover his sight and the most beautiful woman was to be brought before him, he could not determine whether she was handsome or not. Nor if the most handsome and most deformed were produced, could he any better determine to which he should give the preference, having seen only these two."[32]

Be this as it may, it is true that we accept what we are accustomed to more readily than we do the strange or unfamiliar—a fact that helps to explain the wide variations in standards of beauty from one group to another and the antipathy with which deviations from the indigenous standards may normally be regarded.

To test the validity of this statement, we need only go beyond the borders of our own culture. Not only do we find among yellow, brown, and black peoples admiration for their own shades

[29] Ibid., p. 30.
[30] Ibid.
[31] Ross, Edward A., *Social Psychology*. Macmillan Company, New York, 1917, p. 136.
[32] Johnson, Samuel, "The Idler #82," cited by John Callander, *Deformities of Dr. Samuel Johnson*, second edition, J. Stockdale and W. Creech, London, 1783, p. 16.

of pigmentation, or shape of head, eyes, or jaw, and disdain for characteristics that we would consider attractive, but also high regard for certain self-inflicted distortions and scarifications. For example, a common practice among women in East Central Africa has been the extension of their lips with discs until they reach the porportions of saucers. Among some Indian tribes of the Amazon men also follow this practice. Such a bizarre-looking face would in our culture be considered cause for going to the nearest plastic surgeon or joining a freak show. Among the more striking folkways is the Papuans' custom of inserting sticks in the nasal septum (a custom still practiced in several primitive societies), and in New Britain the Arowe mothers' flattening of their infants' heads to give them a sugarloaf shape.[33] The young Thompson Indians of British Columbia used to tattoo their faces to make themselves more pleasing to the opposite sex.[34] A recently discovered stone-age people, the Tasadays of the Philippines, are reported to file their teeth nearly to the gum and blacken them with root juice as beautification, since having full white teeth, they contend, is to "be like an animal."[35] The Hindu hill women of Nepal wear nose rings, and Melanesian women in the New Hebrides have their two upper front teeth knocked out at the time of their marriage to establish their new status. While most people do not carry their ideas of physical enhancement to such extremes, the examples cited are evidence of the vast diversity of the canons of beauty.

Esthetic standards vary not only among groups, but from one period of time to another, particularly in more sophisticated societies. Examples from the past are the fashionably powdered wigs for men in American colonial days, the Heidelberg dueling scars so envied in Germany before World War II, the much admired plump cheeks of the women celebrated in Rubens' portraits, and the hollow Camille-like look affected by American women in the early part of the century. Before Jenner discovered

[33] Mead, Margaret, personal communication.
[34] Tiet, James A., "Tattooing and Face and Body Painting of the Thompson Indians, British Columbia," in *Forty-Fifth Annual Report of the Bureau of American Ethnology*, U.S. Government Printing Office, Washington, D.C., 1930, pp. 403–439.
[35] *San Francisco Chronicle*, July 1, 1971.

his vaccine, a ravaged face pitted by smallpox, which would be of considerable social disadvantage to a woman today, was no deterrent to becoming influential, as was Mme. Pompadour in the courts of Europe. Only recently we have seen some radical changes in American definitions of what is physically attractive and what is ugly. Consider the hippie culture, for example, the popularity of long hair and beards among men of all walks of life and of all ages, and the concept "black is beautiful," which has gone far to reduce the stigma of dark skin.

Several years ago the plight of those who had lost an eye was inadvertently eased by an advertising gambit circulated to promote Hathaway shirts: A black patch placed over the eye of a distinguished-looking gentleman was made the Hathaway trademark. More recently, use of an eye patch by such personalities as Moshe Dayan has practically eliminated its discrediting effect.

Close attention to social forces that have contributed to mutations in concepts of beauty and ugliness provides valuable insight into the nature of attitudinal changes—both rational and nonrational. In the examples just given alterations in attitude were primarily by-products of social phenomena. Two have been outgrowths of ideological movements, (the hippie culture and black power), whereas the vogue of the black patch resulted from a series of fortuitous occurrences (a response to popular symbols and individuals).

While that which is considered beautiful or acceptable varies according to both culture and period, the standards of a particular time and place are more or less defined and fixed. Because no two people look exactly alike, an enormous number of physical divergencies can still meet the esthetic requirements as defined by the given sociocultural norms. But regardless of how wide the range may be, a certain conformity is demanded, and any striking deviation from it plays a decisive role in setting an individual apart. Of the American Indians, for example, the Crow had explicit criteria of personal beauty—a straight nose and skin free of blemishes was mandatory.[36] Similarly, a full oval face was a

[36] Lowie, Robert H., *The Crow Indians.* Farrar & Rinehart, New York, 1935, p. 8.

requisite for Apache girls, while those with big lips, a Roman nose, or a long face were considered ugly. Regarded with equal disfavor was facial hair on Apache men, which they carefully plucked to keep their skin smooth.[37]

The fear of facial irregularities, in whatever form they are defined as such, appears to be universal, and in some societies has been cause for drastic action. In ancient Greece, deformed children were destroyed. The Masai people of Africa, stressing strict conformity in appearance, believed that a child born without a nose or with teeth was a devil who, if allowed to live, would bring down evil consequences upon them. Thus the child was strangled to death; the mother was beaten and the father despised. Among the Hausas of Northern Nigeria the deformed were immediately thrown in the river, and in Borneo their throats were ripped.[38]

It becomes obvious from the examples cited that facial beauty and ugliness, though the concepts themselves may differ, have been and are significant almost everywhere and evoke attitudes that make conformity to the sociocultural norms desirable and, conversely, nonconformity (i.e., ugliness) something to be avoided. Their importance in the value systems of different societies varies in degree, and probably nowhere are they stressed as much and from so many directions as in our own. One has only to consider the immense amount of time and effort Americans spend on their faces to "make a good impression" and win approval. A $7 billion-a-year industry, pandering to and exploiting this high sensitivity to facial appearance, manufactures and promotes blemish removers, wrinkle removers, creams, bleaches, dyes, and the like as aids to the vast numbers of women and men who seek to preserve or improve their status and prestige. The thousands of beauticians, barbers, and cosmetologists—not to mention orthodontists and plastic surgeons—are further evidence of the microscopic attention given to the face and the profound yearning to

[37] Opler, Morris E., *An Apache Life-Way*. University of Chicago Press, Chicago, 1941, pp. 69; 244–245.

[38] Miller, Nathan, *The Child in Primitive Society*. Brentano's, New York, 1928, p. 47.

look attractive.[39] Magazines and newspapers are full of adver-
tisements and slogans with such admonishments as: "You owe it to
your husband and friends to be attractive"; "no one can afford to
look homely or plain"; "dull hair, crooked teeth, or blemished skin
will never find you a job, wife or husband"; ad infinitum. Adver-
tisements for beverages, automobiles, food, and other products
picture glamorous men and women as lures to the buying public,
which not only exalts youthfulness and beauty but likes to identify itself with its models. Even posters used in fund-raising cam-
paigns for the physically handicapped or the mentally retarded
endeavor to create a sensory and an emotional appeal through the
medium of pulchritude. On the other hand, on New York City
subways and buses, an advertisement promoting off-track betting
warns the public against placing bets with a professional gambler
—the gambler being depicted as a sinister man with a large, ugly
nose disfigured by disease.

If we can judge by TV commercials, Madison Avenue, the
public image-makers, and experts in techniques of "impression
management,"[40] the emphasis on external appearance and its
glamorization is so extreme that hardly any other human quality
seems important by comparison. As the role of visual impression
grows, external appearance becomes of major concern. "Expos-
ure" has become a formula for getting ahead, and one's face is his
passport. Since what one sees may take preference over what one
hears, we find that the fate of politicians may hinge upon the skill
of the makeup man—even the President of the United States unabashedly hires professional image-makers to guide him on optimal
cosmetic effects.

[39] Thus the following from eight full pages of an advertisement appealing to the consumers of beauty, with pictures of beautiful nubile women:
"Coty originates next year's face. The new witty, imaginative face . . .
Coty introduces next year's lips. They're red and plum and bronze and
russet and terrific. Like lips ought to be . . . Coty makes next year's
face and eyes. It's a brighter, vervier, sexier face . . . A warm, intense
little face that's gloss and glowing and alluring in all the right places. . . ."
Ladies' Home Journal, October, 1971.

[40] Term for managing one's conduct, behavior, voice, facial expressions,
etc., in order to give a particular impression. Goffman, Erving, *The Presentation of Self in Everyday Life*. Doubleday, Anchor Books, Garden
City, New York, 1959.

Whether or not one is disturbed by the apparent superficiality of our values—by contrivances to gain votes, to make money, or to gain partisans of an opinion—we are dealing with a social fact, one well known to readers of *The Selling of the President 1968* to have played a major part in the strategy of Nixon's campaign advisers. At the time of the now famous Kennedy–Nixon debates, it was claimed by many that Nixon's "five o'clock shadow," which had not been concealed from the TV audience, contributed in no small measure to the poor impression he made. Following that salutory experience and convinced of the need to make their candidate "glamorous and honest," one of the speech writers put it bluntly: *"Response is to the image, not to the man. . . .* It's not what's *there* that counts, it's what's projected—and carrying it one step further, it's not what *he* projects but rather what the voter receives. It's not the man we have to change, but rather the *received impression."*[41] "A candidate's appearance and demeanor," concludes Gene Wyckoff in his study of political campaigning on television, "appear to provide viewers with the most substantial clue to his character. The rational import of what the candidate says . . . appears to have very little influence on the viewers' perception of image."[42]

The seemingly successful efforts of the mass media to conceal or disguise the visible imperfections of the prominent and would-be prominent has given impetus to a growing public to demand the same for themselves. Many people, confusing plastic surgery with a form of magic, have come to believe that getting their faces "changed" is the answer to their life problems. Both men and women, frightened by the onset of middle age and its signs, in order to maintain jobs, sex appeal, or prestige, go to doctors who will "lift" their faces or remove wrinkles or double chins. At the same time this urge to look young and glamorous has opened the way for a flourishing but dubious practice in the field of cosmetic surgery by the ill-trained and unscrupulous. The results are sometimes tragic, as in the case of a 27-year-old man who was fearful

[41] McGinniss, Joe, quoting Raymond K. Price, *The Selling of the President 1968*. Simon and Schuster, New York, 1970, p. 31.

[42] Wyckoff, Gene, *The Image Makers*. The Macmillan Company, New York, 1968, p. 217.

that his career as a singer would be hampered by the dark circles under his eyes. Treated by a "specialist in the correction of facial defects," whose name he saw in a newspaper advertisement, he was interviewed by us two months later. The skin on his face had been so severely burned by the treatment that it was questionable whether or not it would ever regain its normal appearance. Such catastrophes are not uncommon and are further testimony of the coerciveness of the sellers of beauty.

In societies, then, where high social and economic value is placed upon physical beauty and where it has become, as in our own, a dominant cultural interest as well as a saleable commodity, a deformity or disfigurement of the face holds profound social and psychological import for the affected individual.

CHAPTER THREE

Living with a Deviant
Face: Disfigurement,
Identity, and the Self

RESPONSE TO ONE'S SELF[*]

> . . . I hated the streets. In all the diffident,
> casual glances there were hidden needles bear-
> ing a corrosive poison, though those who had
> never been targets could not be expected to
> understand. The streets quite exhausted me.
> I felt like an oily dustcloth, covered with
> shame.
>
> (Kobo Abé, *The Face of Another*)

Considering the increasing amount of research on the social and
psychological problems of those with physical disabilities,[1] it is of
singular interest that so little attention has been given to the
facially disfigured or deformed members of our society. Perhaps
this is in part because of a tendency to think of the "physically
handicapped" in terms of physical limitations, and, when compara-
tive judgments are made, to minimize the deprivations of the
facially crippled because they are presumably able-bodied and can
perform the basic tasks of daily living. This assumption carries a
special irony, for as studies have shown, to the nonhandicapped
facial disfigurements are among the most anxiety-producing and
least tolerated of all types of visible physical disabilities.[2] In addition, conspicuous defects of the face, particularly those involving

[*] See Notes at back of book.

[1] For extensive bibliography of studies on these subjects, see R. G. Barker,
B. A. Wright, L. Meyerson, and M. R. Gonick, *Adjustment to Physical
Handicap and Illness: Social Psychology of Physique and Disability*. Social
Science Research Council, Bulletin 55, New York, 1953, and Wright,
Beatrice A., *Physical Disability—A Psychological Approach*. Harper and
Bros., New York, 1960.

[2] Safilios-Rothschild, Constantina, *The Sociology and Social Psychology
of Disability and Rehabilitation*. Random House, New York, 1970, p. 128.
See also Richardson, Stephen A., N. Goodman, A. H. Hastorf, and S. M.
Dornbusch, "Cultural Uniformity in Reaction to Physical Disabilities,"
American Sociological Review, vol. 26, no. 2, 1961, pp. 241–247.

the mouth, eyes, and skin tend to provoke esthetic rejection and strong feelings of aversion that exclude intimacy or extended interaction.[3] Even when the facial defect is slight or the total configuration is only mildly atypical, unfavorable reactions by others are common, although perhaps more covert.

It is true that except when disfigurement is accompanied by some functional impairment, as in the case of a harelip with a cleft palate, the physical activities of the facially disfigured are not restricted. Their difficulties, like those of minority group members who exhibit traits that are seen as stigmata and are socially visible, reside almost entirely in the social and psychological implications of their particular type of deviance. This is because an individual's ego is validated through the eyes of others: Much of how one feels and behaves, his identity, the image he has of himself is related to the perceptions, assessments, and expectations of others in face-to-face interaction. If, as is generally the case, he is devalued or receives differential treatment because he looks different, the most serious consequences of his deviance will be social and psychological. A demonstration of this is provided by the results of a study of 115 plastic surgery patients made by the writer from 1946 to 1949.[4] Both clinic and private patients[5] were interviewed during a three-year investigation of the psychosocial aspects of facial deformities. (See Table 1) The number of interviews varied; some patients were seen for as many as fifteen hours, others for three. The majority were followed postoperatively for periods of from two months to three years.

---

[3] *The Structure of Attitudes Toward the Disabled*, Brief. Division of Research and Demonstration Grants, Social and Rehabilitation Service, Department of Health, Education, and Welfare, Washington, D.C., vol. 4, no. 6, December 15, 1970, pp. 1–4.

[4] Macgregor, Frances Cooke, "Some Psycho-social Problems Associated with Facial Deformities," *American Sociological Review*, vol. 16, no. 5, 1951, pp. 629–638.

[5] Study of clinic patients was financed from 1947–1948 by a research fellowship from the Manhattan Eye, Ear and Throat Hospital, New York City. The opportunity to interview private patients was made possible through the generous cooperation of Dr. John M. Converse.

An exploratory study prior to the above was made in 1946–1947, the results of which are incorporated in "The Sociological Aspects of Facial Deformities," unpublished master's thesis. University of Missouri, 1947.

TABLE 1
*115 Plastic Surgery Patients According to
Age, Sex, and Marital Status*[a]

	SEX		MARITAL STATUS		
AGE (YEARS)	MALE	FEMALE	SINGLE	MARRIED	DIVORCED OR SEPARATED
Under 15	6	7	13	—	—
15–20	13	11	24	—	—
21–30	22	22	36	8	0
31–40	12	11	12	8	3
Over 40	1	10	4	6	1
	—	—	—	—	—
Total	54	61	89	22	4

[a] 74 were clinic patients; 41 private

The facial defects ranged from gross to mild from the surgical standpoint and were classified according to origin of complaint as congenital, traumatic, pathological, surgical, familial, and cultural.[6] Some patients' faces were so misshapen by trauma or disease that original appearance was almost obliterated; there were greater numbers whose complaint was one conspicuous feature such as a scar, a malformed nose, or protuberant ears. It was observed, however, that the severity of the disfigurement was in no direct proportion to the degree of phychic distress it engendered nor the kind of adjustment made to it. Each case was unique, and such factors as family, social setting, and personality configuration not only differed in each instance but played important roles in the victim's attitude toward his affliction and the type of adjustment he made. Regardless of the difference either of degree of deformity or personality structure and environmental factors, however, the group had many common problems. These centered

[6] The classification *cultural* has been employed by the author to define those cases in which plastic surgery is requested for the purpose of changing an inherited physical trait, usually the nose, which identifies the individual as a member of a particular ethnic or cultural group. When the deviation is the result of a congenital malformation or familial trait, but plastic surgery is requested because the possessor feels the feature identifies him with a group to which he does not belong, the case is also classified as cultural.

mainly around society's attitude toward the atypical face, the low value placed upon it, and the concept of self, which is largely derived through social interaction.[7]

While the age range was from 1½ to 43 years, the table shows that all but 24 of the 115 patients were between the ages of 15 and 40, a period in which the need to be physically attractive is particularly urgent. The greater number of patients was between 21 and 30, a time when jobs and marriage, if not already attained, become major concerns. With a facial defect, both these goals become difficult, often impossible to achieve. The impact of this realization is one of the principal reasons for most of the elective plastic surgery in this age group.

The complaints of the majority of patients centered around the interaction between themselves and others. Not only were they daily dismayed by the reflection in their own mirrors, but, more damaging to their self-image and ego esteem, they saw their handicaps reflected in the reactions of others toward them. These reactions, as noticed by patients and which they stated made them self-conscious and unhappy, were: stares, remarks, curiosity, questionings, pity, rejection, ridicule, whisperings, nicknames, and discrimination. Thus, a girl of 20 with a facial paralysis said she noticed that people looked over her shoulder when they talked to her. "This makes me feel self-conscious. It's as though they didn't want to look directly at me. They think if they do that I'll be embarrassed so they think they're doing me a favor by looking over my shoulder. I'd rather have them look at me—my eyes—back and forth, yet not stare." She complained that children mimicked her expression and made funny faces—especially when she was in school and attempting to recite.

Besides the shame and humiliation caused by such manifesta-

---

[7] Mead, George H., *Mind, Self and Society*. University of Chicago Press, Chicago, 1934, Part III. The more recent formulation of Erik Erikson presents ego-identity as developing out of "the complementarity of an inner (ego) synthesis in the individual and of role integration in the group." "Identity, Psychosocial" in *International Encyclopedia of the Social Sciences*, vol. 7, 1968, p. 61. However, in depicting identity as a social construct, Erikson, unlike Mead, pays great attention to the individual's physical development. *Identity, Youth, and Crisis*. W. W. Norton, New York, 1968.

tions of disapproval, major problems confronted the patients in their attempts to find employment, attract members of the opposite sex, or make friends. Set apart as different from others, rebuffed, and even regarded as social outcasts, they frequently became psychologically disturbed, an outcome that was often far more serious than the actual physical impairment. Most patients suffered from disturbances ranging from feelings of inferiority, shame, self-consciousness, frustration, preoccupation with their deformity, hypersensitivity, anxiety, and more severe manifestations were paranoid complaints; and partial or complete withdrawal from social activities, antisocial behavior, and psychotic states.

CONGENITAL DEFORMITY

The following case history illustrates a succession of manifestations in a man who suffered all his life from the reactions of others to his marred face.

Tom M. had incurred a birth injury that resulted in paralysis of the right side of his face. When in repose his defect, though noticeable, was not dramatically disfiguring. His left eyelid drooped slightly and did not open or close completely when he blinked. When he spoke, however, his handicap became most conspicuous: He literally talked out of the side of his mouth. If he had not had a facial paralysis, he would have been considered good looking. He was slim and well built, had nice eyes, good skin and hair, and was neatly dressed, well mannered, and intelligent.

Tom came from a middle-class family of Irish-American background and was the eldest of five children. His father, a policeman, managed to support his family fairly comfortably. In Tom's infancy his parents noticed that when he cried or laughed he "screwed up" one side of his face. But not until he began to talk did they realize the seriousness of his affliction. They took him to many doctors, all of whom said nothing could be done because the facial nerves and muscles had atrophied.

Upon entering school Tom soon learned that something was "wrong" with his face. "It was my teachers who first made me self-conscious," he said.

> They would stop me in the middle of a recitation and ask me what was the matter with my face. They would say, "Try and control it and don't talk on one side of your mouth like that." This embarrassed me because I couldn't help talking the way I did. In trying to help me they crossed me up by mentioning it in front of the other children. If they had only waited until after class was over!

Tom came home from school promptly every day, not lingering on the streets with other children, who had begun to taunt him—"I became self-conscious and shied away from everything and everybody. I hung around my mother in the kitchen. She taught me to cook and did everything she could think of to keep my mind off myself." The only children he occasionally played with were the "fireman's kids." "I liked them because they had a brother who had a clubfoot and they never mentioned his deformity or mine."

In high school Tom's life was similar to days in grammar school. He preferred poor grades to the teasing of other students. He did not try to make friends nor did he participate in school dances or other social activities. Out of school, he said, he was "driven" into sports to prove that he was a good ball player, "so the fellows in the neighborhood would overlook my face." But when they played other teams, their opponents would try to upset him by calling him "Crooked Mouth" or admonishing the batter to hit (the ball) back at him and "straighten out" his crooked face. This upset him so much that he would leave the game.

When Tom was in high school his mother died, and he decided to leave home and school and go to work. "But I was always given jobs where I wouldn't meet people . . . so it didn't help much." Though his ambition was to be a policeman like his father and grandfather, when he applied he was turned down. "They gave no reason, just said I failed the physical." Later a friend told him the physician refused to pass him because of his deformity.

Tom then tried to get a job in a department store. Six times he was rejected but eventually, through the intervention of a friend, was given work in the packing department where he would not be seen by the public. This job, like all subsequent ones, presented difficulties. "The fellows made my life miserable. They would tell jokes and make faces the way I do when I talk. Or they would say, 'Are you trying to be tough, talking out the side of your face?' "

Though just 18 and earning a small salary, Tom married the only girl he had ever dated. She lived in the same neighborhood and he had known her since he was 10. In high school they went together, "usually to the movies where I wouldn't be seen or stared at." She was the only girl who didn't make him feel uncomfortable about the way he looked, and he was devoted to her. He wanted to get married and "have responsibilities so that I wouldn't feel that life wasn't worth anything." At first he was opposed to having children, afraid they too might be deformed. Nevertheless, three children were born. As each came, Tom anxiously watched for signs of the defect with which he was afflicted. Meanwhile he worked hard at odd jobs to keep his family together on the small salaries he was able to make. "I always have to go for jobs where they'll take anybody."

When seen at the plastic surgery clinic, he had lost his last job because "business was slow." There had been an opening in the company for the position of salesman, which he wanted but didn't apply for because he knew he'd be turned down. "My handicap has made me feel so inferior and afraid to compete with others that I don't dare try. Besides, I can't express myself to the boss or fight for something because when I get nervous my face gets twisted more than usual and I can't be myself." Instead, he accepted a job as superintendent of an apartment house in order to obtain an apartment for his family.

When not working, Tom spent his time at home with his children. He avoided all outside contacts because he couldn't tolerate the staring of others or the quick, furtive glances toward and away from his face. This self-imposed isolaton resulted in some "serious arguments" with his wife, who was very sociable. Tom said:

I just can't enjoy myself when I go anywhere, even with my wife's relatives. If I laugh my mouth goes sideways. It dampens everything for me. I get embarrassed when I talk, and so I don't say anything. Other people seem repulsed by my appearance or embarrassed when they talk to me. It seems like they want to get away. If I go anywhere I always hear people off in a corner saying, "What's the matter with him?" If they asked me outright it wouldn't hurt so much.

In addition he noticed the way they unconsciously drew up their mouths in imitation of him while watching him talk.

They don't seem to realize that it's not my fault that I look this way, and one crack about my face stops me cold. I will go home and brood for two months and draw into a shell. I get cross and snap at the kids and my wife and won't talk to any of them.

The year before, Tom had gone to an eye clinic because his eye was irritated from his inability to close it completely. He was referred to the plastic surgery division with the suggestion that he might receive further help. His hopes, suddenly raised, were as rapidly shattered when he was told corrective surgery was not possible. "For the first time in my life I went out and got drunk," he said. The following summer he drove 2000 miles, mainly in Quebec, to visit, among other shrines, that of St. Anne de Beaupré, "hoping for a miracle."

At the time of our initial interview, a year later, Tom had returned to the hospital clinic. He had heard of a new surgical technique for facial paralysis and hoped there would be some chance for him.

My relatives said the doctors might use me for a guinea pig and I'd only be worse off than I am now. But I'd rather take a chance. I can't be worse off than I am and even if it fails, if by having the operation I can help someone who comes after me, I'm glad to do it. I'm filled with pent-up emotion; I can't laugh or smile or do anything. I have long periods of depression and resentment. I'm terribly sensitive. Even in the movies if I see another handicapped person I get tears in my eyes faster than a woman. I've been so handicapped all my life, so ridiculed and humiliated, that anything is worth trying.

Again the doctors told him that in his case surgery would be of no avail.

Tom said even though there seemed to be no hope for him, he was going to have his son's lop ears corrected. "The kids are beginning to call my son 'Rabbit Ears.' I don't want him to go through what I have."

While Tom made a relatively good adjustment to his life situation and was able to marry and support a family, he was crippled psychologically. His feelings of inadequacy and his periods of depression were caused less by his deformity than by the anticipated and actual reactions of others to his appearance. Being given derogatory nicknames by his peers, offered jobs where he would have a minimum of social contact, and characterized as "tough" accentuated behavior patterns of a negative nature. Not only did his own feelings of frustration and deep hostility prevent him from developing more favorable aspects of emotional life, but his personality distortions were in turn projected upon his environment. His periods of depression, short temper, and refusal to enter into social activities distressed his wife and children and disrupted the family harmony.

FIRST REACTIONS TO ACQUIRED DISFIGUREMENT

For everyone with a marred face there is always a moment of truth when there comes the shocking realization that one's face is "different." Tom, born with a facial anomaly, learned the truth when he went to school. The older child and the adult, who suffer a traumatic change in appearance after years of living with a certain conception of their looks, often learn the truth in one searing moment. Consider the case of Charlotte:

Charlotte B., age 36 and divorced, had suffered for a prolonged period from frontal headaches. It was discovered that she had chronic suppurative frontal sinusitis. A radical operation involving removal of a large portion of the frontal bone resulted in a deep, conspicuous depression in the midportion of her forehead, and a scar across her nose. When she saw herself in the mirror, she was so distressed that she cried for two days. She would not let any of her friends visit her: "I felt I would look so repulsive to others," she said. After two weeks the swelling and inflammation had subsided, and the wound looked less disfiguring. Her courage somewhat restored, she returned to her stenographic job, which she had held for seventeen years. Before two weeks had passed, her self-confidence was severely undermined. "People continually asked me questions and stared at me—in the office, in elevators. Even in buses and public dressing rooms, strangers looked at me and asked what had happened." When she resumed her work after office hours as a nurse's aide in a hospital, an activity she had thoroughly enjoyed, the patients questioned her so much about her disfigurement that she felt unable to stay. "My friends tried to cheer me up by saying, 'It's not very nice to look at, but some-day you can have it fixed.' "

Until her operation Charlotte had been sociable and outgoing. She loved to dance and play bridge with friends, but afterward she refused to go anywhere. "I couldn't stand the staring." She had a "steady boyfriend" but would no longer go out with him. She declined to meet new people because it made her so nervous and self-conscious. She learned to avoid the eyes of others by turning her head or keeping it down and she bought dark glasses to cover the nasal scar. Her depression and preoccupation with her appearance deepened, and she spent many hours weeping. As her anxiety increased, she began using barbiturates and on several occasions had considered taking "the whole bottle."

Charlotte's doctor had told her that in a few months plastic surgery could be performed. To earn enough money she tried to get a job in a restaurant after her regular office hours. "But I was always turned down. They would look at my face and say they had no position available."

Eight months later, when seen at the plastic surgery clinic, Charlotte was filled with self-pity and was semihysterical. She appeared to have lost all interest in dress and grooming. "If I had known the results of this operation," she wept, "I wouldn't have had it. I have wished many times my headaches were back and not this awful disfigurement. It's nerve-racking to be stared at and asked questions all the time, and it makes me want to slap people in the face."

She felt she couldn't "go on" unless something was done to correct her appearance. She was afraid she would lose her job because of her inability to concentrate, and she felt she could never get another one because of her looks. She was also frightened by the thought that she would no longer attract men. "I want to marry again some day and this defect would certainly interfere."

Charlotte underwent reconstruction of her frontal bone by grafts removed from the ilium. The results were highly successful. At the end of three weeks, except for a slight scar, her face appeared to be normal. She herself was remarkably changed. In contrast to her former drab and untidy appearance she was well groomed and her expression radiant.

> I've been a different person since this operation. It's as though I had gone to sleep and awakened as somebody else. I look in the mirror and grin from ear to ear and spend hours looking at myself. Before, I couldn't bear to see myself. Everyone is amazed at the physical and mental change in me and I feel relieved of a great weight. I've gone out with my boyfriends and to parties and restaurants almost every night since I got home from the hospital. I don't cry anymore, or feel inferior; I'm glad to get up in the mornings.

Charlotte's case shows the rapidity with which social and psychological conflicts may develop when a facial deformity is acquired. It resulted in complete alteration of her personal relationships with consequent severe damage to her self-esteem. Deep-seated personality distortions were not incurred, which might not as easily have been removed as the physical disfigurement, because of the short time she was forced to live with it. Her self-concept had been challenged but not permanently altered.

The cases of Charlotte and Tom, just cited, show the social and economic cost of prejudice against one with a conspicuous or unesthetic defect, and how it can play a powerful role in determining his attitude toward himself and his mental health. The facial cripple who experiences years of being shunned or who is regarded as a curiosity or a sterotype is deprived of the security of group acceptance. Judged as different, receiving differential treatment, he may come to believe he *is* different or inadequate and, accepting the identity, may behave in accordance with others' appraisals of him. Conflict between social opportunity and inner desires may arouse frustration and anxiety. Enforced awareness of one's affliction saps both time and energy. To relieve anxiety, to compensate, and to devise coping techniques require efforts that might otherwise be directed toward more positive aspects of living.

COPING TECHNIQUES AND FACE-SAVING STRATAGEMS*

While this writer's studies have shown that each patient's reaction and adjustment to his handicap were unique and depended upon such factors as age at onset of the deformity, parental handling, personality structure, and duration of deformity, those patients with noticeable defects did share many problems traceable to the responses of others, already discussed. Major difficulties most frequently mentioned were related to employment, making friends, opportunities for marriage, and discrimination in various forms. But patients also found, when in public places or social encounters, that the humiliating and erosive effects of violations of privacy, such as staring, remarks, and questions, or obvious eye avoidance, were particularly devastating and sometimes even more demoralizing to their dignity and sense of worth.

The coping techniques of patients and the forms of adjustments they made varied according to the individual and his particular situation. Some were relatively adequate, others resulted in greater maladjustment, but all patients endeavored by one method or another to reduce the strain generated by their appearance. There were those who tried to avoid difficult situations by remaining aloof. Some shunned certain types of social activity, others sought as much seclusion as possible. To cope with unsatisfied needs and

* See Notes at back of book.

feelings of anxiety and insecurity, some patients became markedly aggressive. Others blamed extrinsic factors, such as parents, the environment, or society for their frustrations and failure to succeed. Some patients used their deformities as a defense against hidden emotional disturbance.

A more covert method of adjustment—one the patients themselves were unaware of—was revealed by an interdisciplinary study of 74 patients[8] in which they were asked to evaluate the severity of their deformities according to the scale: slight, moderate, marked, or very marked.

Of the 46 patients who so judged themselves, 22 were classified by the staff as being in the marked or grossly deformed groups. Twenty of the 22 classified themselves as less severely deformed than the staff did. This seems evidence that the severely disfigured, if they attempt to function in society (and all 20 of these patients were doing so), feel impelled to deny to themselves and/or others the reality of their appearance. At the other end of the scale, the staff evaluated 10 patients as having slight deformities, but 7 of these considered their defects to be either "moderate" or "marked"—in other words, more conspicuous than they were in the eyes of others. The psychiatrist diagnosed 5 of these as borderline schizophrenics, and the other 2 as more maladjusted than the group as a whole. In all 7 cases, therefore, the evidence is that feelings of inadequacy in the personality were transferred to the physical defect, which in turn the patient put forward as the cause of the maladjustment.

Patients also revealed a high sensitivity to the differentials in attitudes toward the genesis of deformity and the symbolic meaning accorded it. In our society, congenital malformations or those caused by or suggesting disease, are generally viewed with disapproval. On the other hand, a prizefighter's saddle nose or a war wound may, in certain situations, be more acceptable— indeed may have prestige value. If the deformity suggests a socially discredited origin, the patient appears to be influenced by it, as are the reactions of others. Many patients are careful to draw

[8] Macgregor, Frances Cooke, Theodora M. Abel, Albert Bryt, Edith Lauer, and Serena Weissmann, *Facial Deformities and Plastic Surgery: A Psychosocial Study*. Charles C Thomas, Springfield, Illinois, 1953.

the distinction themselves as to the acquisition of the defect in order to avoid the unfavorable reactions they anticipate. A university instructor always made it a point to explain that an accident had caused his recently acquired facial scars. Although no one had ever implied as much, he was afraid that people would think he was an ex-convict.

Misconceptions and misinterpretations on the part of the beholders about the origin of a deformity are sometimes so tenaciously adhered to that patients have difficulty correcting them. Among our cases was a 56-year-old seaman who had incurred partial avulsion (a forcible tearing or wrenching away) of the end of his nose when he was being attacked and robbed. The lacerations were sutured but required time for healing before plastic surgery could be undertaken. In the interim it was necessary for the patient to resume his work, and he went to sea with a crew he had never seen before. The men asked him what kind of disease he had and inferred that it was cancer. When he told them he had been a hold-up victim they did not believe him, and he was forced to produce a medical certificate to prove it—"The fellows then apologized, and from then on, I was accepted."

Some patients learn through experience that it is advantageous to hide the origin of their deformity, for if they tell the truth they become objects of pity and fear.

Because of an extensive tumor a 48-year-old woman underwent resection of the right half of her lower jaw. The operation left a deep indentation in the side of her face. She grew extremely self-conscious and depressed about her appearance and, aside from her job, avoided people as much as possible. Three years later, bone grafting restored the mandible, and the appliance temporarily used to hold the jaw and teeth in place left wires protruding from her mouth. As a consequence she had difficulty in eating and speaking, as well as a conspicuous disfigurement. Despite this her mental attitude changed considerably, and she even allowed herself to meet strangers. She said:

I no longer feel self-conscious with people because I am going through the process of correction and know my face will soon look normal. I simply come out and explain that I was in an accident and have had an operation to replace my jawbone. Everyone accepts this and it is perfectly easy. It is better than explaining that I had had a tumor and going into the details of that. Immediately after my jaw was removed I told people that I had a tumor and I could see by their expressions that they felt sorry and didn't want to discuss it. When you mention tumor, people think you have a cancer and will probably die of it. They would change the subject immediately.

For this patient concealing the facts had obvious advantages. Even though surgery temporarily exaggerated her deformity, it provided her with a socially acceptable explanation of her appearance.

Three male patients, aged 6, 13, and 18, each with congenital absence of the ear, manifested some positive behavioral changes once reconstructive procedures were under way. Although they were all required to wear conspicuous dressings or helmets and were questioned about what had happened, they felt much less embarrassed because they could explain they were having an ear operation or plastic surgery. These explanations, they noticed, elicited reactions different from those they had encountered before surgery was started, when they had said, "I was born this way." An operation gave them a certain status among their peers and, in varying degrees, brought the boys a sense of release and more spontaneous social interaction.

When a deformity suggests unacceptable social behavior, the victim is likely to be scorned or ridiculed. A 56-year-old retired police officer, whose nose was disfigured by a tumor, declared that he felt in some ways more "ashamed" and humiliated when his nose was red and bulbous than when it was eventually amputated, because his fellow officers attributed the condition to alcoholism and nicknamed him "Rummy Nose."

Mutilations suggesting assault or self-infliction may produce certain specific reactions. A 38-year-old woman incurred a long longitudinal scar on her cheek when, as she explained it, a man "accidentally cut me with a knife in an attempted attack upon his wife." The patient subsequently refused to return to her job:

I was ashamed to be seen. The scar looks as though it might have been the result of someone's revenge and as though someone must have hated me. I feel when people see it they think I have been in a fight and that I was in the middle of a three-cornered affair.

They're probably saying to themselves, "She probably had it coming to her." I don't feel that people think it's an automobile accident because it's impressed so strongly on my mind how it happened that I feel everyone else knows it too. I once saw a woman
with a scar like this and I thought how terrible for a woman to
have such a scar. Maybe she did something and deserved it. It's
always been on my mind and it goes to show that people don't
always realize what really happened and that it wasn't the victim's
fault.

Since most of our patients were residents of New York City or
its densely populated environs, they of necessity came in contact
with large numbers of strangers and casual acquaintances. When
they went to work or school, as many of them did, on buses,
subways, and streets, they were *seen* daily by hundreds of people.
In brief encounters or exchanges, the individual with a conspicuous facial defect is a stimulus to visual impressions only. If the
latter are false or unfavorable, there is little or no opportunity for
them to be erased or for personality to be revealed.

The "civil inattention"[9] that strangers normally confer on one
another and that makes it possible to move unhindered in public
places and to conduct one's affairs without fear of personal intrusions is denied the disfigured person. Often an object of sidelong
glances, extended scrutinization, "double takes" or "startle" reactions, he feels exposed and defenseless. Since he cannot conceal his
face he has few alternatives for protecting himself against attacks
on his anonymity and the invasions of his privacy. To ward off or
handle these anxiety-producing situations, many of our patients
developed a repertoire of tactics. Which ones a patient employed
seemed to depend upon the particular situation—and this is
extremely variable—and his unique personality. The type of
deformity or its severity appears to have proportionately little
determining influence on the particular mode of response.

Some patients, if stared at or questioned, say they feel helpless:
"What can you do?"; "I just look the other way"; "I pretend I
don't notice"; "I ignore them." Common stratagems used to avoid
being noticed in crowded places, such as the subway or bus, are to
sit in a corner, avert the eyes, look out the window, or bury one's

[9] Goffman, Erving, *Behavior in Public Places*. The Free Press, New
York, 1963, pp. 83–88.

head in a newspaper. Some patients use dark glasses, scarves, or hats as a partial disguise in an attempt to maintain their autonomy and distance from others.

Some patients are defiant and express their hostility when they feel themselves attacked by stares or comments. Many of them report that they stare back at the offenders in an effort to make them drop their gaze. One war veteran said, "I burn two holes through them with my eyes and sometimes I get up and say, 'Well, have you had your fill?'" A 44-year-old woman stated, "When people stare at me, I sometimes get so mad I say, 'Take a good look.'" A 21-year-old man with a residual harelip spoke of his first few days in the navy, which were "pretty tough": "Fellows made wisecracks. Then I took over. I'd wait until I got one in front of a lot of other men; then I'd humiliate him and make him feel ashamed. This technique stopped the remarks from others. I'd lie awake nights figuring out ways to work it."

Patients also dread being questioned about what happened to their faces and handle this in individual ways. One woman stated, "If people really seem interested, I tell them the truth." A young man with facial paralysis said, "If people ask me questions I give them a short answer. I hope they'll get the idea and it will teach them not to ask other people similar questions." A 16-year-old boy with an ear deformity said, "If a fellow makes a crack about my ear, I'll say, 'Look at the hole you've got in your tooth.' No one's born perfect and I can always find something wrong with them." Those whose disfigurements are self-inflicted or incurred under other circumstances that may have stigmatic connotations usually conceal the truth and attribute their appearance to an accident. A 28-year-old man, grossly disfigured by acid thrown in his face, discouraged probing by flippant and sometimes hostile remarks. He varied his replies according to his mood: "I stepped on my face going up the stairs; I was in the war; I put my head up when I should have put it down; I got it for sticking my nose somewhere I shouldn't; I was in a ring wrestling with a bear; I was in an accident. I give them one complete sentence—that stops them."

Some patients with deviant faces have worked out other stratagems for protecting themselves from the effects of having attracted attention, provoked questions, or startled others. A college student with a congenital absence of both ears made a point of getting to his classroom ahead of other students rather than making a late entrance and drawing attention to himself. But when confronted with a situation from which he could not escape, he found that "talking to people fast about their own interests keeps them from noticing my ears so much or asking me questions."

When a disfigurement is so repellent that it generates panic in others, the problem of coping or maintaining one's psychological equilibrium is enormous. One woman, dreadfully mutilated by radical surgery for cancer, whose every contact precipitated a visceral reaction in others, came to face her situation with stark realism:

> When people see something they can't cope with they're in a frenzy and they do and say things that are stupid and foolish. It's their reaction that hurts. They don't realize they're hurting you. It's not their intent . . . but they're stupid and foolish out of being unrealistic. I can't blame them because they've never seen anything like me walking around. Anyone like me is *dead*! I keep thinking to myself, 'Just think how lucky you are. Anyone like you is dead so forget these people. They're unrealistic, they're afraid of their shadows. There's nothing you can do about them. If they don't like it let them cross the street.' They're weak people—that's how I classify them. By classifying them as weak I classify myself as strong and am therefore able to cope with them—which is actually, you know, ego. But this ego helps me.

To establish and maintain social interaction is exceedingly trying for the disfigured and nondisfigured alike in each other's presence. Rituals normally followed in our society in initial interchanges are difficult to observe if there is mutual embarrassment and uneasiness. Such circumstances intensify the omnipresent danger inherent in all encounters—that the nondisfigured will unwittingly cause an affront,[10] and the disfigured will "lose face."[11]

[10] Goffman, Erving, "On Face-Work," *Psychiatry: Journal for the Study of Interpersonal Processes*, vol. 18, no. 3, 1955, pp. 213–231.

[11] The unsettling effect that conversing with a disfigured person has upon many nonhandicapped people is not always nor necessarily caused by the sight of the defect but by the latter's feelings of insecurity about how he should react and how his behavior might be perceived or interpreted, as well as his fear of making a faux pas.

A device employed by several socially skilled patients to reduce strain and embarrassment in first encounters was to make a straightforward reference to their obvious condition. Thus a woman whose face had been scarred by a beauty treatment found it effective upon entering a room full of people to say facetiously, "Please excuse the case of leprosy." This averted questions and shifted attention from her face to the person behind it. Pretending to regard her disfigurement lightly, she hoped others would too; her overstatement prompted them to take a less strong view of it and gave the situation a less personal tone. Similarly, a student who returned to school with his head swathed in bandages following surgery said, "When I get in class I say, 'Oh boy, what a headache!' Everyone laughs and we kid back and forth." Such ploys as these remove from others the burden of feigning unawareness and make for more comfortable interaction.[12] A 37-year-old real estate broker endeavored to minimize the unnerving effect of his gross disfigurement by structuring his confrontations to provide time for his prospective clients to observe him before actual confrontation. "When I have an appointment with a new contact, I try to manage to be standing at a distance and facing the door, so the person entering will have more time to see me and get adjusted to my appearance before we start talking."

While they differ in kind, our patients' overt modes of response have more or less the same function: to ward off feelings of humiliation, shame, or anxiety, and to make the individual feel safer. They fall into three categories: First there is withdrawal or avoidance. By "ostrich" techniques such as hiding, looking away, or ignoring questions, the disfigured try, as it were, to efface themselves in order to cushion their feelings of inadequacy. Such response increases the social distance between themselves and others. The second tactic is overt aggression. When feelings of shame or humiliation are aroused, the patients retaliate by hostile looks or remarks, which, like withdrawal, tend to widen the gulf between them and others, with the deformed face offering an

---

[12] This technique of moving past the initial distance manifested by the nonhandicapped toward the handicapped in order to make one's defect a less crucial factor in social interaction Davis calls "breaking through." Davis, Fred, "Deviance Disavowal: The Managment of Strained Interaction by the Visibly Handicapped," *Social Problems*, vol. 9, no. 2, 1961, pp. 127–128.

initial barrier to satisfactory social interaction and the unfriendly behavior creating an additional obstacle. A third response is that of patients who, accepting the fact that their appearance may startle others, make deliberate attempts to do something about it. By excessive charm, manifestations of friendliness, facetious remarks, or by giving others time to be shocked and to recover, they try to reduce tension and social distance. They offer active responses that, though perhaps veiling hostility, enable them to make contact and to move toward rather than away from people.

Myths and stereotypes, together with the particular personality, the specific situation, and the sociocultural environment determine adjustment to facial deformity. In addition to these variables, the psychosocial data suggest that the consistency of responses to be expected from others plays a determining role in adjustment. A grossly disfigured individual feels that he can almost always count on unfavorable responses, wherever he goes. Seldom, if ever, does he experience immediate approval. Since he expects a negative response, he is usually prepared and will have developed overt or covert techniques of coping with it. There are, however, less conspicuous defects, such as missing ears or facial irregularities that suggest stereotypes, which in certain situations may be laughed at or evoke aversive feelings but under other conditions may be ignored or not even noticed. In general the responses are erratic and unpredictable, and persons with such deformities appear to be in precarious, hair-trigger positions, never quite certain what will happen, alternating between tension and relief. Adjustment to their situation is difficult indeed. In short, predicability and consistency of response permit the grossly deformed to adjust, whereas ambiguity and inconsistency of response seem to aggravate their anxiety. In our studies, whatever form adjustment took, however, each patient experienced some degree of personality conflict and heightened mental and emotional awareness of the self.

To counter the threats and social deprivations of their environment exacts from many patients a high psychological cost. Energies that might otherwise be channeled into constructive endeavors are consumed by wasteful preoccupation with their appearance, vigilant anticipation of the reactions of others, and the building up of defense mechanisms—all of which are detrimental to mental and emotional health.

In addition to the small subterfuges and dissembling by which individuals with disfigured faces seek to protect themselves from the uncivil attention and intrusions of others, there may be more profound responses. Ingrid de Valery, whose story appears in Chapter One, provides an instance of fundamental changes in attitudes and values.

Ingrid's reaction to her transformed appearance was one of defiance. Unlike many other victims of disfigurement, she did not become shy and retiring nor withdraw from society. On the contrary, she forced herself to accelerate her social activities and to engage in economic enterprises involving new forms of interaction. A complex, egocentric, and strong-willed woman, she refused to accept any role inferior to others or to admit defeat. In her efforts to compensate for her deficiency, she developed excessive and emotionalized habits and attitudes that resulted in overcompensation and eventually produced personality distortions that entered into her relations with others. She cultivated her personal assets, both physical and mental, in a deliberate effort to distract from her face. Continually apprehensive about her appearance, she became absorbed in testing her ability to charm and attract others. But her success in doing so did not satisfy her: She wished to control, and, when she failed, she grew angry and childishly vindictive.

Upon material wealth she began to place a value higher than friendship or love and spoke of it as her "compensation for an ugly face," a symbol of power, and a medium by which she could both prove her competence and gain the recognition and praise so necessary to her ego-system. Frankly proud of being "hard and ruthless" in business dealings, boasting, "I am like a gangster," she carried these attitudes over into other relationships.

Because of Ingrid's long-established social position, and her husband's, her disfigurement was apparently no obstacle to acceptance in her group nor did it serve as a barrier to her economic endeavors. Furthermore, a man had married her after she had lost her beauty. These circumstances might have helped to give her some sense of security. But such was not the case. From the reflections of her image in the mirror, from the expressions of pity, curiosity, and repugnance directed toward her wherever she went, she knew she was "different" and set apart. Acutely conscious as she was of her handicap, she conducted herself as though she felt superior, and, resenting manifestations of pity, she endeavored to make people envy her instead.

Prior to Ingrid's accident, the beauty of her face had been a highly visible stimulus to favorable responses from others, particularly from men. Accustomed from an early age to their admiration, she was more or less indifferent to their attentions. But when her face became so tragically transformed this attitude changed radically. She deliberately tried to attract both men and women. Losing interest once she had won a man ("I despise them after they fall in love with me"), she turned her attention to another in order to prove to herself that she was still capable of charming and conquering men and still physically appealing. That she had had numerous affairs helped to bolster her vanity and self-esteem, and boasting of them gave her equal satisfaction. In order to repair the damage to her ego and to tolerate the presence of others, it was necessary for her to find fault with all with whom she came in contact, to play up their real or imaginary defects, and to precipitate quarrels between friends.

In considering Ingrid's reaction to her ruined face and her adaptation to it, one must take into account her Spartan upbringing in which personal defeat as well as physical and moral weakness were inadmissible, and her strong identification of herself with her father, which she fortified after the loss of her beauty by her determination to compete and to win recognition and praise as he had done. She was fortunate in having high status and prestige, which helped prevent her disfigurement from being the social and economic handicap it might otherwise have been. In addition, she was an intelligent, educated, and cultured woman who capitalized on her knowledge of the ways in which she could make herself most acceptable and who exploited them to the fullest.

The social and psychological impact on the disfigured and the methods they use to function in society and at the same time maintain their equilibrium take many forms. As we have seen, some stratagems and coping techniques are more constructive than others in that they make it less difficult to establish relationships and to preserve one's sense of worth. As with other types of disability that are likely to give rise to negative reactions, such feelings as anxiety, pity, threat, guilt, or hostility, which many nonhandicapped persons tend to experience (often unconsciously) in the presence of the disfigured, may be attenuated rather than reinforced by the demeanor of the victim himself—his presentation. That he must bear a double burden—confronting them with his disfigurement and then ameliorating the shock—is a statement not of the way things ought to be but unfortunately, for the present at least, of the way they are.

CHAPTER FOUR

Living with a Deviant
Face: Identity and
Responses of Others

Wandering about the place when Mother was abed and Gideon in the fields, I felt lonesome. I wished there was some shorter way to be as beautiful as a fairy. Then a thought came to me all of a sudden. I wonder it didna come afore, but then I'd never much minded having a hare-lip afore. It seems to me that often it's only when you begin to see other folks minding a thing like that for you, that you begin to mind it for yourself. I make no doubt, if Eve had been so unlucky as to have such a thing as a hare-lip, she'd not have minded it till Adam came by, looking doubtfully upon her, and the Lord, frowning on His marred handiwork.

(Mary Webb, *Precious Bane.*)

"My face is what separates me from the rest of humanity."   (a patient)

INFERENCES AND ASSOCIATIONS*

In the preceding chapter a continuous process of interaction has been discussed chiefly as it is seen in the responses of the disfigured individual. In the present chapter it is presented as manifested in the behavior of others, for identity takes its character in response to the responses of others.

While the complaints and apparent distress of the facially deformed are sometimes viewed with skepticism on the grounds that they are exaggerated, imagined, or projected—and this sometimes may be true—they cannot wholly be discounted. Regardless of whether the patient's complaints are based on experiences or are the reflections of acquired social attitudes, torment and fears

* See Notes at back of book.

become more understandable when we study the attitudes and reactions of the nondisfigured toward those who have physical deviations. That there is a basis in reality for the deep concern manifested by most patients is well illustrated in the responses of a group of nondisfigured individuals to photographs of those with facial anomalies.[1]

One photograph was of a 37-year-old married man whose face had been grossly disfigured ten years before by chemical burns that later developed into skin cancer. Despite frequent hospitalization and his unsightly appearance, he had been able to conduct a fairly successful business as a real estate broker, an occupation that required meeting people daily. Although psychological difficulties were associated with his deformity, his social integration was adequate and he did not entirely avoid going to restaurants or other public places.

No clues were given, yet photographs of his face elicited the following remarks about the cause of his disfigurement:

Was this a war casuality?
Is this syphilis or a physical injury? [The respondent was told it was due to cancer.] Inevitable that the man must be sick in the head, too. Sense of imminent death which comes from this. Close to skeletal impression as you can get. Man so obviously dying and he looks it, too.
Probably a gangster.
Horrible!
Grotesque, inhuman, bad.
A leper.
Looks like an accident.
In a fire or an explosion.

Statements made about the man himself were as follows:

He would have a hard time initially because he is so ugly. He couldn't do anything that would require personal contact. I don't think anyone would hire him.

[1] Post, Rita F., in Macgregor, Frances Cooke, Theodora M. Abel, Albert Bryt, Edith Lauer, and Serena Weissmann, *Facial Deformities and Plastic Surgery: A Psychosocial Study*, Charles C Thomas, Springfield, Illinois, 1953, p. 101. Similar results were attained in Jørgen Hviid's study, *Reactions of the Non-Handicapped Toward the Handicapped*. Gyldendalske Boghandel, Nordisk Forlag A.S. Copenhagen, Denmark, 1972.

Such an extreme kind of deformity must have a terrific effect on practically all people, so a person like this would have one hell of a time getting any satisfaction in social situations and probably would tend towards isolating himself as much as possible both from society and the gaze of other people.

Oh God! I wonder how he remained alive at this point. It's horrible! It proves that his urge to live is terrific if you can live with that face. Naturally he lives in seclusion. What does he do for a living? I certainly don't think he does work with any people. Probably does some kind of work by himself. Probably digs ditches or is a writer. He must have a tremendous interest in life. Seems to me he would want to destroy himself.

When he has to go out in public he does, but only under the most severe compulsion. He couldn't get a job.

Another photograph was of a 31-year-old man of superior intelligence, a junior executive in a chemical corporation. Because of congenital malformation, his facial contours were asymmetrical and incongruous: a low, narrow forehead; a prominent, convex nose; a receding, pointed chin; narrow, deepset eyes; large buck teeth; lop ears. He was classified as markedly deformed. Of 60 respondents, all but one reacted unfavorably to his picture. Thirty classified him as mentally inferior, 27 as "lethargic," "dull," "weak," "dazed," and only one judged him as a "nice, quiet man." His combination of facial features in our society seemed to symbolize a definite stereotype. The following conclusions were drawn about him:

He is mean and small—not bright.
He looks mean and nasty.
He might be a follower in a gang.
He's a dope addict.
I wouldn't hire him for a job where he would meet people because I think his appearance is against him.
Man seems to look like a maniac. Has desire to kill.
Below average intelligence—probably an IQ slightly above or even in moron group.
Repulsive because of deformed teeth.
Appears to be an imbecile; very low intelligence.

Another markedly deformed subject, age 29, had strabismus and a saddle nose. A soft-spoken young man, he had studied to be a teacher but later went into business. Judgments based on impressions received from his picture were as follows:

This guy looks like the real criminal type.
Tough baby.
Looks like a boxer from the shape of his nose.
Looks ignorant. Reminds me of a pug.
Nothing malicious-looking about him, but not the kind of guy I
    would like to get into an argument with.
One-track mind.
Laborer.
Slightly moronic.
He's stupo. He's an ex-navy gob and hangs around a poolroom.

It is interesting that these three patients had managed to function far better than the respondents anticipated. Although all had serious social and psychological problems connected with their deformities (one was, in fact, receiving psychotherapy), they had achieved relative economic success. Equally striking is the high percentage of unfavorable emotional response (repulsion, fear, contempt) and of cultural stereotyping (subnormal intelligence, low social and economic status, moral turpitude). Facial features that served as false clues led respondents to impute to these patients not only socially unacceptable personality traits but inferior roles and statuses as well. In short, the marred face may debase identity.

The widespread prejudice surrounding the facial cripple, which the responses so vividly reflect, does indeed exert pressures that are difficult for him to cope with. While these must not be minimized or passed over—on the contrary they must be thoroughly understood if he is to be helped—it is of the utmost importance that they be related properly to any psychological disturbances he may have. All too often such disturbances, regardless of their etiology, are attributed directly to his deformity: "It is no wonder when he has such a terrible handicap." Conversely, if he achieves a modicum of success, people are surprised; they anticipate personality difficulties that would preclude it. These attitudes are not confined to the uninformed but may be found in upper social and educational brackets, as illustrated by the following examples:

After corrective surgery one of our patients described her pre-operative appearance to a prospective employer. The latter listened sympathetically and then remarked, "It's a wonder you did not become an alcoholic or a lesbian."

The teacher of a 12-year-old patient who had a residual scar from a harelip operation explained the child was the shyest one she had ever had. "I know it [the deformity] has made her shy. She sits dreaming about her lip—I know it from her expression. . . . She has very poor marks—I do not think because of lack of intelligence, but she does not concentrate. She is too involved in her thoughts about herself."

A staff conference was held with a vocational adviser regarding a 19-year-old girl whose severe psychological disturbance stemmed from her unfortunate family situation. Although she was distressed over the sequelae of a harelip operation, this played a relatively unimportant role in her basic disturbance. The vocational adviser, however, insisted that it was solely because of the facial defect that the patient was maladjusted and had been rejected by her family and friends. She added with finality, "Anyone who has a facial disfigurement has a terribly difficult time." Furthermore, the adviser discouraged the girl from pursuing her ambition to become a nurse on the ground that she would automatically be rejected because of her appearance.

A well-educated businesswoman whose husband had incurred a nasal deformity during World War I insisted that it was because of his sensitivity about his damaged appearance that he committed suicide twenty years later, although substantial evidence pointed to other causes.

The above examples illustrate the assumption on the part of so many that any behavior disorders present in those with facial deformities are caused by the defect alone. That the deformity may have been a causal factor, or an accompaniment of other circumstances and pressures, is seldom thought through. There is a strong tendency to oversimplify, to explain on a direct cause-and-effect basis, and to evaluate the personality of the facially disfigured not only in terms of appearance ("he is the criminal type") but of presumed psychological concomitants ("he is mean-tempered and dishonest").[2] As a consequence, socially created images of the deformed often become distorted reflections of their personalities, which can significantly control their behavior and social adjustment. Such individuals often not only must make personality adjustments to their distorted reflections but are sometimes impelled to behave in a manner expected of them, although it be contrary to their basic needs and desires. This in turn may produce severe psychological conflicts and make adequate adjustment difficult, if not impossible.

STEREOTYPING

As has been noted, the problems of the facially deformed are complicated by the fact that the appearance of the face, or a feature of it, is often endowed by others with particular personality or character traits (in our culture a high forehead, for example, is supposedly an indication of superior intelligence). This phenomenon, known as social or cultural stereotyping, works to the disfavor of those with facial deviations. For them, prejudgments are usually derogatory, even stigmatizing, tending to hamper satisfactory social interaction. The type rather than the severity of deviation seems to call up these responses. A man with a low forehead or a receding chin—both mild anomalies—is apt to be written off as deficient in intelligence or weak in character. In a milieu where racial or religious prejudice prevails, a large convex nose, the Jewish stereotype, may automatically assign to its possessor all the physical, mental, emotional, and moral characteristics with which that group is supposedly endowed. Other facial deviations tend to evoke laughter and ridicule. Large, protuberant ears and noses of conspicuous size or shape suggest caricature, and

[2] The same mechanism may operate conversely when the deformity is corrected or removed. The patient may find that the moodiness and short temper that used to be excused are no longer tolerated; those about him fail to realize that the disfigurement was only one factor, in many cases, in a long history of unhappiness and maladjustment.

our patients with such defects almost unanimously complained of being the butt of nicknames, jokes, and outright amusement. The faces of other patients suggest even more discrediting identities—gangster, moron, drug addict, or one afflicted by a dreaded disease (cancer, leprosy, syphilis). The ubiquity of many of these stereotypes can be attributed to folklore, literature, television, and movies, in which the unsightly face is utilized as a visible symbol or a personification of evil, disease, criminality, or mental deficiency.[3] In any event, the popular mind may use these identifications, in one way or another, as a springboard for a generalization: An unsightly face is an accurate portrait of the character and personality behind it. Such misconceptions and interpretations seem to play a significant part in the sense of self, the self-regarding attitudes, and the subsequent development of psychological conflicts in many of the facially deformed. The force and prevalence of these social attitudes also account in great measure for the strong emotional reactions that often appear to be disproportionate to the patients' specific defects. The following statements of some of our patients, suffering from congenital or traumatic defects, express their dread that others will assume that, as a result of the defects, they harbor undesirable characteristics:

Patient with a harelip and cleft palate: "Children would make fun of the way I talked and looked and said I wasn't normal."
Patient with saddle nose: "I'm always being asked if I'm an ex-prize fighter."
Patient with facial paralysis: "People think I'm a tough character because I talk out of the side of my mouth."
Patient with grossly disfigured face due to war injuries: "When I parked my car in front of a jewelry store, two cops came up and asked me for my identification card. They thought I was a gangster."
Patient who incurred a marked deformity due to radical surgery for cancer: "People seem to think I've changed because my face has."

[3] Even those with scientific training are sometimes influenced by a deeply entrenched emotional quality which obscures their intellectual objectivity. For example, an anthropologist told of interviewing an American Indian who had a facial paralysis; and while he recognized the affliction for what it was, he couldn't overcome his feeling that she was not "quite on the square" because of her distorted mouth. Macgregor, Frances Cooke, "Some Psychosocial Problems Associated with Facial Deformities," *American Sociological Review*, vol. 16, no. 5, 1951, p. 631.

Patient with gross congenital malformation: "I avoid restaurants as people may think I have a disease and won't want to eat after me."

Even disturbed patients who fixate on some facial feature appear to utilize social attitudes and stereotypes to reinforce their fantasies, although the defect of which they complain is often imaginary. They insist, "people are laughing at my big nose," or "people think I lead a dissipated life because of the bags under my eyes." Though such cases have obvious psychiatric implications, the social forces that foster and perpetuate these attitudes and the cultural conditions that provide the setting for these specific interpretations must be taken into account.

Stereotyping of Dentofacial Defects*

On those whose deformities evoked ridicule, bordered on caricature, stimulated jokes, and were sources of amusement, the psychological impact was exceedingly great. In fact, many patients with such deviations were in worse psychological states, exhibited more behavioral disorders, and were more maladjusted than those with deformities that were distressing to look at or tended to elicit strong emotional reactions such as pity or revulsion. For individuals suffering from dentofacial defects this is often the case.

The person with buck teeth ("Bugs Bunny Syndrome") or a receding chin is less apt to be viewed with compassion than as a target for teasing, nicknaming, or caricaturing. As Aristotle said, the thing at which we laugh is a defect or ugliness that is not great enough to cause suffering or injury, and thus a ridiculous face is ugly or misshapen, but is one that suffering has not marked. Yet, to the victim, derisive laughter is one of the most devastating instruments men can use, and the shame, anger, and distress it can generate are immeasurable. Such reactions to derisive laughter appear to be universal. Some societies, the Sioux Indians for example, well aware of its effectiveness, have deliberately employed ridicule as their most potent weapon for keeping an individual in line.[4]

---

* See Notes at back of book.
[4] Macgregor, Gordon, *Warriors without Weapons*. University of Chicago Press, Chicago, 1946, p. 116.

No one knows nor can know how many lives and personalities of those with noticeable malocclusion and dentofacial disfigurement have been adversely affected in past generations. We do, however, have some knowledge of persons who have reported and spoken of suffering from particular problems in this connection. In her writings Eleanor Roosevelt described her feelings about being what she called an "ugly duckling." She had a miserably unhappy childhood and young adulthood, and had to struggle long and valiantly before she succeeded (overtly, at least) in overcoming her shyness and feelings of inferiority. (Would she have become the great person she was had she not had this visible handicap?) During her years as First Lady, caricatures of her were legion—always with large protruding teeth. Late in life she finally had relief: In an automobile accident she lost three or four of her front teeth. Following dental restoration she remarked with unabashed delight what a fortunate accident it had been, because at last she had straight front teeth.[5]

Even in the absence of stereotyping, there are two other handicaps associated with dentofacial deformity. The first is that the area in and around the mouth is both emotionally charged and strongly connected with one's self-image. As an instrument of speech, eating, and kissing, as well as a mirror of emotions, it also has unique social and psychological implications and symbolic meaning. Any abnormality in this area, therefore, is not only highly visible and obtrusive but, as research has shown, tends to evoke a type of aversion that is both esthetic and sexual.

The second handicap is that such defects interfere to a greater or less degree with the flow of social interaction. The man without an arm can partially hide its absence in a sleeve; a cripple in a wheelchair can attend a dinner without generating uneasiness. But the same cannot be said of those with facial defects. Because in normal interaction the eyes attend the face, any irregularity can be distracting and produce uneasiness for the afflicted and the non-afflicted alike. Spontaneous interaction requires certain skills and rules on the part of both participants. But spontaneity is inhibited by the rule of "not noticing." Not to notice dentofacial irregu-

5 Roosevelt, Eleanor, personal communication.

larities is especially difficult, for, as Goffman notes, "the closer the defect is to the communication equipment upon which the listener must focus his attention, the smaller the defect need be to throw the listener off balance. These defects tend to shut off the afflicted individual from the stream of daily contacts, transforming him into a faulty interactant, either in his own eyes or in the eyes of others."[6]

SOCIAL AND CULTURAL STIGMATA: MOTIVATION FOR PLASTIC SURGERY OF THE NOSE[7]*

Reducing visibility by changing names or by altering physical appearance for the purpose of eliminating a characteristic that sets one apart from others is of particular interest to the social scientist for the insights these types of behavior may provide into such phenomena as assimilation, stereotypes, identification, and conformity. In the case of immigrant and minority groups in the United States, both methods have been employed in attempts to solve problems of marginality and assimilation, and to adjust to the dominant culture. For example, the anglicizing of surnames has been a common practice since the early days of colonization.[8] Negroes have long used skin-whiteners and hair-straighteners, whereas American Indian and Asian women, by permanent waves, seek to "correct" straight hair. In these instances steps are taken

---

* See Notes at back of book.

[6] Goffman, Erving, "Alienation from Interaction," *Human Relations*, vol. 10, no. 1, 1957, p. 53.

[7] The material on which this paper is based was collected in a larger study on the psychosocial aspects of facial deformities, which was supported in part by a grant (M-201) from the National Institute of Mental Health, United States Public Health Service, and by the Milbank Memorial Fund. For the opportunity to analyze these data I am indebted to The Association for the Aid of Crippled Children.

[8] For detailed discussion see H. L. Mencken, *The American Language*, fourth edition, Alfred A. Knopf, New York, 1938, pp. 474–505. Also Leonard Broom, et al., "Characteristics of 1,107 Petitioners for Change of Name," *American Sociological Review*, vol. 20, no. 1, 1955, pp. 33–39.

to reduce "differentness" by disguising traits that in an Anglo-American society are familiar clues to group identity.[9]

Another device for reducing visibility is cosmetic rhinoplasty—a surgical procedure for altering or reshaping noses that are considered unesthetic or that have symbolic significance. Although social scientists have given attention to physiognomy as a clue to ethnic background and group membership,[10] they have virtually ignored the phenomenon of nose alteration as a means to an understanding of the heavy pressure that society brings to bear on its members to conform to the "American look."

One explanation may lie in the prevailing assumptions about people who might seek plastic surgery for other than gross nasal disfigurement. Quickly expressed, they are as quickly dismissed as obvious. For example, those most likely to have "nose jobs," as they are popularly called, are commonly thought to be:

Women more than men, because "women are vain."
Entertainers and models more than those in other occupations.
The well-to-do more than those in middle or low income brackets.
Jews more than non-Jews, because they want to "pass" as non-Jews.
"Neurotics" more than "average" or "normal" people.

What follows is a report of a study of 89 patients who requested cosmetic rhinoplasty, aimed at shedding light on the social and cultural components of their motivation. Because of the nature of

[9] When there is a rise in national pride, the need felt by individuals or groups to disguise their ethnic origin may be dissipated. For example, with the growth of Italian nationalism under Mussolini, name changing by Italian-Americans virtually halted. (Mencken, op. cit., p. 493.) More recently a comparable reversal is to be found among young American Negroes. With the advent of the African independence movement, a new sense of identification has awakened among Negroes who were formerly anxious to conceal their racial origin. As a consequence the market for hair-straighteners and skin-whiteners has declined. (*Time*, 83:26, Jan. 3, 1964.) Also of interest is the substitution of the letter X by Black Muslims for English surnames inherited from the days of slavery.

[10] See, for example, Allport, Gordon W., and Bernard M. Kramer, "Some Roots of Prejudice," *Journal of Psychology*, vol. 22, 1946, pp. 9–39; Scodel, Alvin, and Harvey Austrin, "The Perception of Jewish Photographs by Non-Jews and Jews," *Journal of Abnormal and Social Psychology*, vol. 54, no. 2, 1957, pp. 278–280; Savitz, Leonard D., and Richard F. Tomasson, "The Identifiability of Jews," *American Journal of Sociology*, vol. 64, no. 5, 1959, pp. 468–475.

the population, some of the findings may be unique; hence no claim is made to representativeness or generalizability. The major concern here is with the implications of the findings, the questions they raise, and the clues they may provide to further investigation.

The data were collected in New York City from 1946 to 1954. Sixty patients were from the plastic surgery clinic of a voluntary hospital and 29 from a plastic surgeon's private practice. They were first seen by a plastic surgeon, then interviewed by me. Originally I saw all who requested rhinoplasty; eventually such patients were selected on a nonsystematic random basis, determined by available time. Interviews averaging three to four hours per patient were conducted both pre- and postoperatively.[11]

In their initial consultations with the doctors, some patients tried to conceal their real motives by complaining of functional impairments, such as a deviated septum, nosebleeds, or frequent colds.[12] Men more often than women were reluctant to admit concern about appearance and resorted to the more socially sanctioned motive of a physical disorder. But in interviews with me, such patients eventually revealed that their primary motive was appearance because they contemplated surgery only if it included correction of the visible defect.

Another stratagem the patients used to conceal their motives was a statement about esthetic requirements for jobs in the entertainment field, although there was no evidence that they were otherwise qualified for such work.

Common complaints of the patients were the "appearance" of the nose and the social and/or psychological handicap they felt it to be. All perceived it as a source of distress that would be alleviated by surgery. Deviance was defined as a nose that was "too big," "too long," "flat," "twisted," "humped," "bulbous," "retroussé," "hooked," "disporportionate," "ugly," or identifiable with a minority. Some patients attributed the shapes of their noses

[11] Except with 18 patients who were advised against or decided against surgery.

[12] External deformities are often combined with a deviated septum, which can impair breathing. Excluded from this series of patients were those whose noses were marred by partial loss, skin damage, or growth processes caused by disease.

to congenital malformations, to accidents, to surgical failure, or to heredity.

A striking item (Table 1) is the proportion of male patients: 49.4 percent. In American society preoccupation with appearance is expected of women, and rhinoplasty is becoming socially sanctioned. But in men, until very recently, surgery of the nose motivated solely by vanity was suspect. Although no data are available on the total number of men and women in the population who undergo cosmetic rhinoplasty, this study indicates that men make up a larger percentage of them than is commonly supposed.

Although the findings do not support the assumption that show people and the rich are more likely than others to seek cosmetic rhinoplasty, the internal differences in the series do not necessarily negate it. Had a Hollywood surgeon's patients been studied, the occupational distribution might have been different.

TABLE 1
Age, Sex, Marital Status

		NUMBER	PERCENT
AGE	16–19	21	24.0
	20–29	46	51.0
	30–39	15	17.0
	40–46	7	8.0
	Total	89	100.0
SEX			
	Male	44	49.4
	Female	45	50.6
	Total	89	100.0
MARITAL STATUS			
	Single	64	72.0
	Married	14	16.0
	Divorced, separated, annulled	10	11.0
	Widowed	1	1.0
	Total	89	100.0

Similarly, with respect to income there is no claim that these figures could be generalized to the whole population of rhinoplastic patients. Private patients with higher incomes represented but a fraction of the total number of nasal plastic patients seen by the surgeon during the period of the study. The larger proportion of clinic patients, 67 percent, is accounted for by the fact that I saw more clinic than private patients.[13]

While this series may not be representative of the total population, the findings do indicate that dissatisfaction with appearance and desire for surgical intervention are not restricted to members of any one occupational group nor necessarily to the wealthy.

From Table 2 one might infer that the better educated are not so concerned with physical defects as the less educated. Since most of the subjects were clinic patients, they were a lower socio-economic, hence less educated, group. Despite this apparent distortion, the wish to alter the nose seems to be independent of the amount of education.

As Table 3 shows, the greatest number of patients were second-generation Americans. As to religion, the ordinal position of Catholics, Jews, and Protestants is the same as that in New York City's population as a whole. Of the Catholics, the largest ethnic group represented was Italian—22 patients or 61 percent—of whom 21 patients were second-generation Americans. Despite the large number of Irish Catholics in the city, only 3 of the Catholic patients were of Irish extraction. The balance had their national origins in such diverse countries as Lebanon, Armenia, Portugal, Greece, Russia, Argentina, Germany, Denmark, and France.

Of the Jewish patients, 60 percent were second-generation Americans. The same proportion were of East European background and the rest mainly from Austria, Hungary, and Germany.

Six Protestants were second-generation Americans of Italian, Greek, Czechoslovakian, Armenian, or Syrian background.

To summarize the social and cultural characteristics of the 89 patients: (1) the majority were young single adults of both sexes; (2) they were largely in occupations other than professional and

---

[13] Admission to the hospital as a clinic patient was based on income.

TABLE 2

Occupational Status, Income, Education

	NUMBER	PERCENT
OCCUPATIONAL STATUS		
Professional, proprietor, managerial	9	10
Sales, clerical	20	23
Skilled	8	9
Semiskilled, service, unskilled	21	24
Housewife	11	12
Student	19	21
Armed Forces	1	1
Total	89	100
INCOME		
High	10	11
Middle	26	29
Low	52	59
Not ascertained	1	1
Total	89	100
EDUCATION		
Postgraduate work	3	3
College graduate only	2	2
Some college	16	18
High school graduate only	21	24
Some high school	38	43
Elementary school only	6	7
Not ascertained	3	3
Total	89	100

managerial and were predominantly of upper-lower and lower-middle socioeconomic status; (3) most had not gone beyond high school; (4) they were mainly first-, second-, and third-generation Americans, and Catholic or Jewish. While the data are statistically inconclusive, they do suggest that the stereotyped portrait of those who seek rhinoplasty is at variance with the facts in many respects.

TABLE 3

Immigrant Status, Ethnocultural Background, Religion

	NUMBER	PERCENT
IMMIGRANT STATUS		
First-generation American	8	9
Second-generation American	56	63
Third-generation American	13	15
Old White American	3	3
Negro American	1	1
Non-US citizen	6	7
Not ascertained	2	2
Total	89	100
ETHNOCULTURAL BACKGROUND		
Jewish	33	37
Italian	23	25
Armenian, Greek, Iranian, Lebanese, Syrian	9	10
American (Old White 3; Negro 1)	4	5
Austrian, German	4	5
Irish	4	5
Polish, Russian	3	3
Other	9	10
Total	89	100
RELIGION		
Catholic	40	45
Jewish	31	34
Protestant	10	11
Other	4	5
No affiliation	4[a]	5
Total	89	100

[a] The statements of two of these patients were interpreted as a repudiation of their parents' religion, which was Jewish. However, when Jews are discussed as an ethnocultural group in this study, these two patients are included.

Motives

What are the reasons underlying patients' unhappiness with the appearance of their noses and their requests for plastic surgery? Study of this question has been made for the most part by psychiatrists, psychoanalysts, and plastic surgeons. For understanding of patients' motivation these specialists have focused their attention

largely upon preconscious and unconscious factors. Their interpretations have centered around symbolic castration; conflict in
sexual identification and ambivalence in patients' identification
with parents[14]; the symbolic (sexual) meaning of the nose and the
wish for surgery[15]; concepts of body image, and neuroses and
psychopathology among patients.[16] Although some reference is
made to social and cultural factors that on a "conscious" and "realistic" level "seem" to be instrumental in decisions to seek surgery,
attention to these elements has been superficial. This is of singular
interest, in view of the attention given to the nose throughout
history. Not only has it been considered an index of character and
in certain instances of racial and ethnic identification, but probably more than any other single physiognomic trait it has been
stereotyped, value-laden, and the butt of countless jokes.[17]

To slide over the role that social and cultural factors may play
in determining the wish for surgery and to concentrate on the
more deeply rooted psychiatric factors is to obscure and by
implication to oversimplify two other important dimensions: the
relationship between the patient and his social and cultural milieu,
and the extent to which our society brings pressure to bear on its
members to conform to its standards.

Although conflicts in sexual identification, ambivalent identifications with one or both parents, and various degrees of psychic
disturbance may, on an unconscious level, be of "central importance" in many patients' quests for surgery, concentration on these
interpretations can limit our understanding. There are other con-
ceptual frameworks that can provide perspectives and interpretations of this phenomenon. One of these involves the concept of
social perception and the role of the face in human interaction

[14] Meyer, Eugene, W. E. Jacobson, M. T. Edgerton, and A. Canter, "Motivational Patterns in Patients Seeking Elective Plastic Surgery, I. Women
Who Seek Rhinoplasty," *Psychosomatic Medicine*, vol. 22, no. 3, 1960,
pp. 193–201.

[15] Friedman, Paul, "The Nose: Some Psychological Reflections," *American Imago*, vol. 8, no. 4, 1951, pp. 3–16.

[16] Linn, Louis, and Irving B. Goldman, "Psychiatric Observations Concerning Rhinoplasty," *Psychosomatic Medicine*, vol. 11, no. 5, 1949, pp.
307–315.

[17] Holden, Harold M., *Noses*. World Publishing Company, Cleveland,
1950.

and identification. Within this theoretical framework the nose may be considered as distinctive a mark of an individual's identity as his name. If, in addition, the nose is atypical, as a social stimulus it is a significant deterrent of a person's social and psychological situation.

Crucial to understanding the motives of persons who decide to alter their noses is an examination of their stated reasons. The statements of the patients in this study have a certain validity and explicitness that reflect both social values and the degree to which these are perceived as creating problems for the deviant. I do not discount the inferred meanings in their statements, but I am less concerned here with the "deeper" psychological implications than with the social and cultural determinants.

The complaints of the majority of patients centered on their patterns of social interaction. Emotionally they were affected by the reactions of others, such as stares, remarks, avoidance, ridicule, and nicknames. These led to preoccupation with appearance, feelings of inferiority, shame, depression, hypersensitivity, resentment, and so on. Economically and socially their major problems were obtaining jobs, getting ahead, making friends, and finding marriage partners.

Such were the difficulties that characterized the group as a whole. On another level, there was a distinguishing feature that separated the patients roughly into two groups.[18] This was related to the specific nasal deformity. Here was found a significant difference in its socially symbolic meaning for and effect upon the patient and those he encountered. In Group One, ethnocultural considerations and group stereotyping played a predominant role; in Group Two, individual interpretations and personality stereotyping were major problems.

Group One. The "Changers."

Of the 46 patients in Group One, 59 percent were Jewish; most of the others were Italian, Armenian, Greek, Iranian, and Leba-

---

[18] With the exception of 8 patients whose statements were too obscure for classification in either group; and of these, 6 had severe psychiatric disorders.

nese. These patients believed their noses identified them with certain ethnic or religious minorities. They wanted their noses "changed." The particular contours with which they found fault were for the most part replicas or variations of what physical anthropologists refer to as an "Armenoid" nose: one characterized by considerable length and height, convexity of profile, a depressed tip with a downward sloping septum, and thick, flared alae or wings.[19] Although not characteristic of all Jews,[20] the Armenoid nose or modifications of it is a feature of many Jews, Armenians, Syrians, Greeks, Turks, and other Levantine peoples.[21] It is also common in parts of the Mediterranean and in Eastern Europe.[22] While the exaggerated convexity of the nose is far from being universal among Jews—more typical are the recurved and flared nostrils—it has nevertheless become stereotyped and caricatured in Western society as a "Jewish nose" and selected as a symbol that differentiates Jews from non-Jews.

Interviews with Group One patients revealed that on a conscious level prejudice and discrimination—real or imagined—with all that these imply played an important role in their wish for surgery. Common complaints were being referred to by terms identifiable with minorities: Jew, hebe, wop, dago, guinea, and Greek. These persons wanted to "look like an American," a statement to which some Jews added, "I want a turned-up Irish nose."[23] In other words, they were primarily dissatisfied with their noses as visible clues to an ethnic or religious group that they perceived as having unfavorable or stigmatic connotations which they could eliminate by surgery, simultaneously achieving an appearance that would more nearly conform to the majority's.

[19] Hooton, Ernest A., Up From the Ape, rev. edition, Macmillan Company, New York, 1947, p. 518.

[20] It has been said that the "Jewish nose" is present in only about 15 percent of adult Jewish males in New York City. Huxley, Julian S., and A. C. Haddon, We Europeans. Harper and Bros., New York, 1936, p. 149.

[21] Hooton, op. cit., p. 518.

[22] Shapiro, Harry L., The Jewish People: A Biological History. UNESCO, Paris, 1960, p. 71.

[23] Perhaps because of the large Irish population in New York City, Irishness is viewed by some minority group members as synonymous with being American.

The largest number of patients in this group were Jews (27). Typical of the reasons they gave for requesting surgery were:

Male student, age 18. I'm not afraid to admit I'm Jewish—in fact I'm proud of it. But competition is very rigid here in America. I want to fit into the social pattern. My nose is a hindrance with girls. I want to conform so I won't have to conform.

Seamstress, age 45. If you're Jewish-looking you don't stand a chance, or if you have a Jewish name you don't stand a chance, either. There's too much competition in the business world.

Female bookkeeper, age 21, a Sephardic Jew. I am taken for Yiddish by Jews. I feel the stereotype Jewish nose is like mine. I don't mind saying I'm Jewish, but when they look at my nose and say it's a "Jewish nose" I don't like it. Spanish Jews have straight noses. They say my nose looks "Yiddishm." I want to look typically American. You see a typical American and she turns out to be Irish, so I guess that's what I want.

Female typist, age 25. I feel I am just as American as anyone else, but my nose sets me apart and keeps me from feeling I belong. [My friends] have modern faces, not a nose that shrieks your nationality. When I'm with Gentiles I feel a curtain comes between us because of my nose. It identifies me as Jewish. . . . I want to look like an American.

Male secretary, age 29. In the merchant marine I met anti-Semitism. I was called a "Jewish so-and-so"—a "Jew with a circumcised nose." I don't want to feel as though I have the Palestinian map all over my face. I don't talk with a heavy accent, or go to a synagogue, or show my jewelry to the world, but my nose is a hindrance.

Pressure brought to bear by others was instrumental in the decisions of several Jewish patients to request surgery.

College student, age 24. (This patient's parents had urged both her and her brother to have surgery. Her mother said: "My husband wanted our son to have a nasal plastic. You know my husband is downtown in the garment district, and lots of people there have it done. He told the boy, 'You have to have a good appearance when you meet new people. You'll see it will pay.'") Said the patient: People in the garment district say, "When are you getting yours done?" All of them are nose-conscious down there. I don't want to have anything to do with them. I'm anti-Semitic—I think most Jews are. It's hard to be a Jew. People have such strange ideas about them, as though they're not really human.

Female model, age 18. I want to get ahead so badly, yet I'm stopped at every turn because I have a Jewish nose. If you notice in *Harper's Bazaar* or *Vogue*, all the girls have little turned-up noses. . . . I changed my name . . . but the first photographer I went to said, "You changed your name but not your nose, didn't you?" Another said, "You can't have your race written all over your face if you want your picture in fashion magazines."

Female secretary, age 24, refugee. I'm proud of being Jewish and always tell people I am. A change in my nose would not hide the fact that I am Jewish. My friends here say it would be better if I had it changed, and I would have better opportunities for jobs or friends. In coming to the United States, my nose is evaluated as a defect by others. I hadn't thought of it before.

Several patients initially were guarded about their reasons for wanting surgery but in postoperative interviews spoke more freely. Though delighted with the results of his rhinoplasty, an 18-year-old high-school dropout at the same time admitted to deep anger: "I have had my nose changed due purely to the fact that I live in a society where there are conventional forms to follow. The pressure to conform and the discrimination is too great."

Five Jewish patients were less specific. Although they made oblique references to looking "Jewish," concern about it was either brushed over: "I never met discrimination—only when I was little," or denied: "Not because my nose was Jewish, but because it hooked downward." These patients, as did many other Jews, referred to friends or relatives who had had a "nose job" or a "nose bob," saying: "Everyone is having it done—it's a fad."

The 19 non-Jews in Group One were also concerned with identity problems related to ethnicity and religion. Seven of these patients were Italians, all of whom were Catholic. Typical statements were:

Male wood finisher, age 26. I've been kidded in school and in the army—called "hook," "beak," "guinea." A nasal plastic operation would make me look less foreign. They think I'm French or Greek. I would like to look more American.

Female candy wrapper, age 42. Everywhere I go people take me for a Jew. It doesn't bother me, though. I like Jews and I like working with them. But I'd just like to be taken for an American. . . . It's been hard for me to get jobs because employers ask me if I'm a Jew. I have to talk Italian to convince them.

Housewife, age 22. I'm always taken for Jewish in the Italian neighborhood. I wear a cross so people will know I'm a Christian. I want to look like a Catholic.

Male merchandise marker, age 21. I need to have my nose changed. I've been called "wop," "guinea," "dago," "spaghetti bender."

An 18-year-old delivery boy wanted his nose "changed" not only because he rejected his Armenian heritage—"who wants to be one?"—but because "people always think I'm Jewish."

A 37-year-old Iranian of Moslem faith, the wife of a physician, said:

I want to beautify myself. I only thought of it since I came here. In Persia we don't care. Persians have Aryan blood. Most people here think I'm an Italian Jew or a South American Jew. It doesn't bother me if people think I'm a Jew. I have not this prejudice. I just want to look better. Since I've been here I've met many Persians and Europeans who had it [rhinoplasty] done. There is more prejudice about Jews in Persia, but we are not taken for Jews there. They know better the characteristics of the face and by the way you talk. Their [the Jews'] accent is different. We can tell the difference. Here, as a foreigner, people can't distinguish between us. Everybody thinks this is a Jewish nose.

For two patients, elimination of racial characteristics was the main issue. One, a 29-year-old model, wanted her broad, flat nose narrowed and straightened. She said: "I don't find it advantageous to have decisive Negro features. The less you look like a Negro, the less you have to fight. I would pass for anything just so long as I'm not taken for a Negro. With a straight nose I could do costume work and pose as an Indian, Egyptian, or even a Balinese."

The other patient, a 24-year-old bookkeeper, had inherited slant eyes and a flat nose from her Filipino father. She wanted to eliminate part of her "oriental" appearance and believed rhinoplasty would do this.

Group Two. The "Fixers."

Of the 35 patients in Group Two, 33 (92 percent) were non-Jewish, of whom almost half were Italian. The major considerations of Group Two patients were related to individual rather than group identity: Of critical importance was the relationship between the high visibility of an unesthetic facial feature and the impression it gave to others. The total effect evoked by an unsightly nose not only elicited negative reactions but, patients reported, often led to false perceptions and distorted images of their personalities and characters.

The nasal defects characteristic of Group Two patients were of three types: congenital malformations, idiosyncratic family traits, and disfigurement caused by trauma. Represented were noses that were crooked, concave, flat, bulbous, retroussé, asymmetrical, had deflected or cleft tips, and were abnormally large or long. As contrasted with patients in Group One, who wanted their noses "changed," Group Two patients wanted their noses "fixed." Or, in cases of recently acquired deformities, patients anxious to recapture their original appearance wanted their noses "repaired." Unlike those in Group One, who wanted to become "Americanized," their aims were of a different order. They wanted to be identified as "what I *am*—not what I look like" and to avoid the social and psychological handicaps of ugliness in a society whose cultural bias toward beauty, youthfulness, and conformity is extreme.

As victims of the generalized prejudice against physical deviance, Group Two patients were subjected to staring, comments, teasing, jokes with sexual connotations, caricatures, and nicknames. Such humiliations were held responsible in large measure for precipitating or reinforcing great dissatisfaction with themselves and the way they looked. The labels applied to them were highly individualistic and stylized. Suggested resemblances to birds, animals, fruit, and to persons whose noses had become social stereotypes had earned them such names as Polly, The Hawk, Falcon, Little Moose, Banana Nose, Tomato Nose, Pinocchio, Cyrano, Durante, and Bob Hope. Other equally descriptive terms were Beak, Schnozzo, Hook Nose, Split Nose, Tweedlebeak, Ski Snoot, Punchy, and Pug. Patients said such appellations, whether facetious or not, caused them extreme embarrassment, distress, and/or resentment. And in the light of these some patients reported a "reflected image phenomenon"—"It's gotten so that when

I look in the mirror I don't see what I see—I see what they say."[24]

Negative reactions to a particular shape of nose as a symbol of certain behavioral or personality characteristics were frequently experienced by those whose appearance resembled social stereotypes. These led to distorted images and expectations, to which several patients had found themselves almost forced to adjust.[25] "Because I look like a clown, people expect me to act like one." Indeed in some instances the image became the "real thing," and the patient not only adopted but exploited the role assigned to him. For example, a 35-year-old man whose nose resembled Durante's had spent half his life as a professional comedian, having discovered that as long as he played the comic he was "able to get along."

In several cases situational factors played a predominant role in motivating patients to seek surgery. A former boxing instructor had not found his saddle nose a liability in his job as a physical education teacher. But when he joined a finance and loan company, the stereotypical traits imputed to him proved to be a handicap. In his initial contacts with clients, references were made to his being a "fighter." Such gibes as "Do they send you after me if I don't pay the loan?" became irritating. He requested rhinoplasty so he wouldn't "feel like a ruffian" in a job where he had to meet the public.

The discrepancy between what was suggested by the nose and the person himself was a source of distress to most Group Two patients. Unique was the longshoreman, aged 18, who viewed as an asset the false image his flattened nose provided. Looking "tough" while working on the docks was useful. "The fellows think I'm a boxer. They're scared of me. Even the girls seem

[24] If, as Cooley says, "we live with our eyes upon our reflection," this act can be a two-edged sword for the facially deformed, who obtain an unfavorable conception of their appearance not only from the reactions of others but from the mechanical reflection as well. Cooley, Charles H., *Human Nature and the Social Order.* Schocken, New York, 1964, p. 247.

[25] For an excellent discussion of the function and consequences of stereotyped images in human relations see Gustav Ichheiser, "Misunderstandings in Human Relations: A Study in False Social Perception," *American Journal of Sociology*, vol. 55, no. 2, part 2, 1949, pp. 26–56.

impressed with the idea that I'm a boxer." He had come to the clinic only after an employment agency had urged him to have cosmetic rhinoplasty if he wanted to change his occupation.

In contrast, a 24-year-old bus driver whose nose was also flattened sought surgery because he objected to looking like a fighter. "In general the public don't think much of a boxer. They think he's tough and illiterate. In the movies the boxer is always a dope. I couldn't even be a waiter—I look too tough."

Some patients felt that they were regarded as objects rather than as persons. A bricklayer, aged 25, wanted to have his nose reduced in size. For years he had suffered the humiliation of being called "The Nose" and introduced to girls as "Big Nose." Even though he was recognized for his athletic prowess, such remarks as "The Nose is scoring again" had driven him to leave high school. Unable to tolerate the constant embarrassment, he had withdrawn from all social contacts. Desperately anxious to "get a girl and get married," he finally borrowed money from friends to finance an operation.

The patients' extreme sensitivity about their noses was on several occasions made more explicit following surgical correction. Self-concepts too painful to discuss prior to surgery were revealed, once the stigmatic trait had been removed. A 19-year-old female bookkeeper said, "Before the operation I looked like an ex-con. Now I feel as if I'm part of the world again."

One of the two Jewish patients in Group Two, a 38-year-old businesswoman, requested surgery because for years she had "hated" her looks. "I look like my father. My sisters and mother are pretty. I've resented the fact of external comparisons by others. My reason is pure vanity." The other Jewish patient, a housewife aged 26, had "always admired beauty" and had been self-conscious about her nose as long as she could remember. She was under the impression that it was growing longer.

In summary, requests for cosmic rhinoplasty as a social phenomenon may be seen as a response to socially and culturally defined deviance, and as a reaction to looking "foreign" or "ugly" in a society that values conformity and good looks. In either case, to look "different" or to deviate far from the norm is to be set apart and to receive differential treatment.

In this study patients perceived their nasal deviations as stigmatic and anomalous—as impediments to "acceptability," upward mobility, and achievement of a career or life goals. Plastic surgery was seen as a device by which to surmount the barriers society creates for those who fail to meet its physical standards.

Although there were multiple and overlapping aspects in the motivation of patients in Groups One and Two, certain regularities within each distinguished them. When Group One patients are categorized as "changers," the word "change" implies a change in identity as well as in nasal contour. For these patients the reduction or eradication of ethnic visibility was the predominating motive. Where the nose suggested an ethnic-religious stereotype and elicited prejudice, it was perceived as handicapping. By "changing" it these patients hoped to erase their marginality, merge into the larger culture, and thereby gain acceptance. "Looking American" was in this case identified with becoming "Americanized." The Jews in Group One saw as major determinants of decision to seek surgery religious discrimination, problems of competition, mobility aspirations, and social interaction with Gentiles. To the non-Jews upward mobility and competition appeared to be of less concern than being identified as a foreigner or a Jew. In both instances, however, the basic resolution of societal and cultural problems was ethnic neutrality.

Group Two patients could be described as "fixers." Their requests for surgery may be seen as a response to the belittling attitudes of society toward what is considered physically repugnant, on the one hand, and to the tendency to ascribe undesirable personality characteristics to those with certain stereotypic noses on the other. These patients saw themselves as objects of erroneous projections and judgments and as victims of categorizations that are often made on the basis of a single physiognomic clue. In having their noses "fixed" they endeavored to escape the psychic assaults that result from the discrepancy between "what I look like" and "what I am." In contrast to the "changers," who wanted to change their identity, the "fixers" sought to recapture theirs or to establish themselves as individuals.

In this discussion we can neither ignore nor discount the high incidence of personality maladjustments and/or neurosis that systematic studies by psychiatrists have shown to exist among patients who seek cosmetic rhinoplasty. This study does not call their findings in question. Indeed, it substantiates preliminary findings reported elsewhere that dissatisfaction with the nose is frequently symptomatic of underlying personality disorders.[26]

Taking this into account, we are nevertheless faced with an intriguing question: How can the wide discrepancy between the number of Old White American patients in this particular study population and those of other ethnic backgrounds be explained? Whereas Old Americans may not have the ethnic features characteristic of Group One patients, they are certainly no freer from the kinds of nasal deviations that characterized patients in Group Two. Nor, presumably, are Old Americans more immune than others to personality maladjustments. The hypothesis is suggested that immigrants and members of minorities have certain types of adjustment problems that are not shared by Old Americans. The high visibility of a deviant nose, therefore, is seen as an *additional* handicap that reinforces their marginal position in the sociocultural hierarchy. It is a handicap, however, about which something can be done. Moreover, this requires less effort on the part of the individual than does learning to speak without an accent, for example. Because appearance is an important criterion of "Americanism," altering the shape of the nose may be seen as an attempt to change one's identity as a member of a minority group, as well as an adjustment to the attendant conflicts of an ambivalent cultural identification. Seeking surgery may also be a manifestation of adaptiveness to the American cultural tendency to change rather than to cope, to alter rather than to endure.[27]

Although the problems of Group Two patients were not related to ethnic visibility, it is suggested that members of minorities are

[26] Macgregor, Frances Cooke and Bertram Schaffner, "Screening Patients for Nasal Plastic Operations: Some Sociologic and Psychiatric Considerations," *Psychosomatic Medicine*, vol. 12, no. 5, 1950, pp. 277–291. Also, Macgregor, Frances Cooke, "Some Psychological Hazards of Plastic Surgery of the Face," *Plastic and Reconstructive Surgery*, vol. 12, no. 2, 1953, pp. 123–130.

[27] Mead, Margaret, personal communication.

more vulnerable to dominant group pressure, and looking "conspicuous" or "ugly" is perceived as a problem superimposed upon other problems of adjustment. Even a slightly noticeable defect therefore—to those who are insecure and overly sensitive to their marginal position—becomes intolerable.

It has been observed that the strains resulting from attempts to straddle two cultures are conducive to various forms of neurosis.[28] Thus it might be expected that psychological maladjustment played a significant part in the motivation of many of our patients. There is abundant evidence for this assumption. To better understand the phenomenon of nose alteration, then, we must look beyond the explanations and interpretations found in personality theory and in psychoanalytic and sexual symbolic theory, and examine patients' motivation within a larger context. Regardless of what deeper psychological forces may be operating in the desire to alter one's nose, the wish to do so must also be seen as having its roots in the social and cultural pressures to conform. If the nose did not have symbolic meaning in our society and to those with whom we interact—what direction, we might ask, would the neurosis take? Would the same individuals, except for the occasional psychotic who develops an idée fixe, seek plastic surgery?

As we have already seen, in an environment where prejudice is supported by antipathies toward a certain type of nose, the development of sympathetic interaction is precluded, and the nose becomes a social handicap, which it might not have been in another environment. Similarly, a change of situation or of social setting within the environment can turn a previous asset into a handicap, or the reverse.[29]

---

[28] For examples see Seward, Georgene, *Psychotherapy and Culture Conflict*. The Ronald Press, New York, 1956, and Stonequist, Everett V., *The Marginal Man: A Study in Personality and Culture Conflict*. Charles Scribner's Sons, New York, 1937.

[29] Changes in definitions of beauty can suddenly generate a large-scale demand for plastic surgery. For example, following World War II Japanese women, influenced by American GIs and Western films, began to have surgical alteration of nose and eyes in order to approximate more nearly the Occidental ideal. Similarly the American presence in Saigon has created a trend among both Vietnamese women and men for round eyes and a Western nose, and, for women, dimpled cheeks and larger hips and breasts. *The New York Times*, May 21, 1973.

MYTH AND REALITY

The two following case histories highlight, in part or in sum, essentially the collective attitudes, conflicts, and feelings of the Jewish patients just described, who underwent cosmetic rhinoplasty. Despite particularistic differences comprising their reasons for wanting to "change" their noses and the differences in their histories, there are sufficient fundamental similarities in their problems and motivation to provide two models or "ideal" types. They represent two extremes, the rest of the patients range in between on a continuum.

I'LL BE A GOOD-WILL AMBASSADOR.

Case of Arthur Steelman

Arthur Steelman, age 28, was good looking and well built. He was intelligent, soft-spoken, and mannerly. Though his nose was convex and slightly high, it looked distinguished and in harmony with his face.

Unlike the majority of Jewish patients interviewed, whose initial requests for rhinoplasty seldom included any reference to discrimination or to Jewishness, Arthur was blunt. He had changed his name from Schulberger to Steelman. "It was my first act when I left the army," he said, "because of the fun made of my name. My problem is discrimination. I want an opportunity to make the kind of friends I want." The kind of friends he wanted were Gentiles, and he felt that his nose was a handicap because it served as a stimulus to immediate antipathy and prejudice and precluded establishing satisfactory relationships.

If they had a Shylock on the stage they would give him my kind of nose. I'd like people to like me before they know me. I know I have a good appearance in general, but I can feel people [Gentiles] when they talk to me wondering if I'm a Czechoslovakian or of German background, and trying to place me. They consider Jews foreigners. They try to put me in a category—and Lord help me if I did anything vulgar or loud, or if I cheated. People feel if you're Jewish you must be a rich Jew. If you're not, you must be hiding your money.

Arthur said he did not want others to "wonder" what he was.

I'd rather not have the thing brought up at all. I want them to like me first and then know what I am. It is the intelligent people who look at you that bother me the most. You watch for a smirk or some little thing. The lower-level people are just stupid—but it is the intelligent ones who hurt you and the thing I hate most. I don't want to be hurt any more. Socially and economically I could be strangulated [sic] by this.

Arthur's father was born in Germany, his mother in Austria. He and his older brother and sister were American-born. His father was an insurance agent, and the family lived "comfortably enough" in an apartment in a middle-class, predominantly Jewish neighborhood. Arthur described his parents as being "fairly religious." His father occasionally went to the synagogue but never asked Arthur to go; indeed, the son had never participated in a religious ceremony, but his mother still observed the holidays and "lived by the Golden Rule."

Arthur described his early home life as "unhappy." His father drank excessively and sometimes abused his wife, which infuriated the boy. Because of this situation he formed few close friendships. "If I had friends I could never bring them home. My father was so unreasonable and caused such a commotion, and I never knew when he would kick up. He ruined my whole childhood." Five years before Arthur's surgical consultation, his father had been institutionalized for paranoia.

Arthur had attended public schools where the students were predominantly Jewish and Italian. He said he had kept to himself most of the time since he felt inferior to others because of the situation at home. He had taken no part in school activities but occasionally dated Jewish girls in high school. He was not a good student—"I was always dreaming"—and after three-and-a-half years he dropped out. He took such jobs as errand boy and shipping clerk—"I decided I'd conquer the world."

During this period Arthur first became conscious of his nose. "I just woke up one morning and it was long." Although it was not as long as his father's, there was a close resemblance; it was, in fact, similar to the noses of all the family except his brother's. "His is straight and the only one I admire. I've always admired pretty noses, and I did not like mine." While displeased with the shape of his nose, he did not become inordinately self-conscious about it until he "moved out of [his] own little circle" and enrolled in a drama school. His ambition was to go on the stage, and his studies in this field gave him a "zest for living." He wanted to be in a comedy, but the part called for a "clean-cut American boy," and he "looked like a Roman."

Arthur recalled that he first became aware of "the difference between Gentiles and Jews" when he was about eight years old. His neighborhood included a few Gentiles "of a lower economic class," who often insulted the Jewish children. One day they accused Arthur of "killing Christ." Reflecting upon this experience he said, "You begin to fear at that moment. Jews don't fight —they try to argue their way out, and you are afraid that you'll come to blows." Aside from these early encounters, he said that he had met with no manifestations of prejudice or discrimination during his school years. While working, he made friends with an Irish-Catholic boy whom he admired greatly and with whom he remained a close friend for many years. The boy's mother, however, used to "mock in fun" Arthur's gestures and mannerisms; but it hurt him—"behind the fun there is malice."

Not until he entered the army, at age 22, did Arthur become conscious of his nose as a symbol. There he felt the full impact of being a Jew and the meaning of discrimination. "I got it all the time. Someone was always insulting me. Once two cooks who were drunk began to talk about Jews in front of me and said, 'The Jews are hiding in this war—they don't get killed.'" Arthur said he became upset and angry. "I sent word to my commanding officer that I wouldn't stand for this and that I wanted to see him. But he wouldn't see me, and I thought he was against me, too. In a hotel lobby, when I was in uniform, a fellow pointed at me and said, 'He's a Jew.' If I hadn't been with my friend and fairly conservative I would have hit him. I saw blood."

A Gentile friend was asked in Arthur's presence if he were going to celebrate the Jewish holidays, too. Arthur did nothing at the time, but when the offender appeared in the medical division where Arthur worked the latter "gave him an extra tetanus shot" —"I hated him. It's the lower-level people who are most cruel.

The only defense I have is to be with a nicer type." Although most of his friends were Jews before he entered the army, the friends he made in the service were Gentiles. "I selected them because they fascinated me. My ideal was any good-looking Irishman with a turned-up nose, and I had a burning desire to be accepted." He also dated Gentile girls for the first time. "I never met discrimination with women or felt any animosity from them."

After four years in the army, Arthur was discharged because of tuberculosis. At the time of our interviews he had been convalescing in a sanitarium for two years and now was about to be released. His associates there were Gentiles, and he told of going to see *Gentleman's Agreement* with some of them. "After the movie they were friendly with me and said, 'Now we realize the sort of thing you're up against.' For a few days afterward they acted like decent people, being extra nice and putting themselves out."

Arthur's self-consciousness and growing preoccupation with his nose led him to develop a number of stratagems to hide or distract attention from it. "I dress as well as I can. I always face people 'head-on' to avoid showing my profile. I bought a car too —this is part of it—getting and wanting nice things to make up for my nose."

By the time Arthur consulted the surgeon, his feelings of inferiority had intensified to such an extent that he had begun to withdraw from social life. "I don't like to meet new people, yet inwardly I would love to know them." He felt that for him "culture" was most important—"books, music, and the theater"—and he yearned to know more and to advance himself. To be "cultivated," he thought it necessary to associate with "superior and intellectual people," but felt that his nose prevented their accepting him.

Arthur offered several reasons for wanting a rhinoplasty:

If my nose is changed, I'll be "Jack Armstrong, the All-American boy." I don't want it changed in order to pass for a Gentile, but I just want the subject [Jewishness] dropped. I'm sensitive and easily hurt, and my philosophy now is to stop running. I think people are basically good. If my nose is changed, then I can show them [Gentiles] by my behavior that there are nice Jews. I'll be a good-will ambassador. I can prove to people that I'm not only a "white man" but a "white Jew."

Arthur defined as a "white" Jew one who is liked by non-Jews. He conceded that his affinity for Gentiles had caused other Jews to accuse him of being anti-Semitic; nevertheless, he felt sure that if his nose were changed "people" would be friendly to him. "They will have a chance to know me without prejudgment. Then, when they know I'm a Jew, I will have had time to prove that all Jews are not obnoxious but have good qualities."

His mother did not approve of his desire to alter his nose. She told him, "It's going to hurt you, and if it hurts you it will hurt me. Your nose fits your face. God gave it to you." Arthur's comment was, "I guess she thinks I'm renouncing her and renouncing my faith." She had reported that his relatives were "shocked by the idea," but he retorted, "They're from the Old Country." His friends had said they thought it would change his expression and that he wouldn't be as good looking. Only his brother had encouraged him.

For a week after his operation Arthur wore a dressing over his nose. When the dressing was removed, he looked in the mirror. For a moment he couldn't speak—his eyes widened—he turned pale. Then he exclaimed, "My God! I look like an Irishman! . . . I look like someone I know—and I *like* him, *too*!" Saying that he felt weak, he sat down but rose repeatedly to look at himself. Fascinated, he was examining his nose when his brother arrived. He looked at Arthur, sat down, and—trying to cover his surprise —said measuredly, "It's a good job." Later he said privately to the interviewer, "Now I'll tell you how I really feel. You see, I'm a Jew and I'm not ashamed of it, but it's a shock to have your brother look like an Irishman—not that I have anything against the Irish."

Two weeks later Arthur was in gay spirits and said he was happy with the results.

It's freedom now! . . . I can walk in the streets and look up and down and sideways. I feel free—as though the umbilical cord had been cut 28 years late. Now I'm just an ordinary fellow—not as good looking as I thought I'd be, but I don't mind that. I want to be just an ordinary guy. This business of discrimination is no joke. Did you ever notice the eyes of a Jew? They have the sorrow of 3000 years in them. The damage to the Jews can never be made up.

Arthur said that at home, the morning after the dressing had been removed he had been afraid to look in the mirror.

I had been badly shaken—looking like an Irishman. When I first saw myself I said, "No!"—from the bottom of my feet all the way up. It's like looking in the mirror and having someone else look back at you. A Jew has tremendous pride. That's why it's difficult to get other Jews to admit their reasons for wanting a nasal plastic. It's their pride. I wanted a Jew to know I was a Jew. I didn't want to lose the link with something I was most accustomed to. At the same time I didn't want others to know I was a Jew. At first I was horrified when I looked like an Irishman. I was a man without a country. Now I'm beginning to get used to it.

Arthur said his mother had told him he looked "wonderful," although she repeated that she had been afraid of the operation. His friends at the sanitarium were "amazed." "Some of them couldn't realize I was the same person. They kept staring and I let them. Then, as I talked, they saw I was the same person, and soon they got used to me." He said he was "having a good time" with his new profile. He had asked his "date" if she thought he was good looking. Staring at his profile she replied, "You're cute!" "Before," said Arthur, "I would have driven into a tree."

He felt that he was a "much nicer" person now—"I can tolerate more people. I was nervous before and thought it was the war, but I guess it wasn't. My nose bothered me. I was always running away and procrastinating. I had no confidence and was dreaming all the time." He spoke of plans to return to drama school. Someday, too, he hoped to get married. "I think I'd prefer to marry a Jewish girl. We'd understand each other better. We'd be the kind of Jews they'd like. I'd like to be a philosopher—the kind of philosophic Jew—quiet and wise."

Arthur was willing to have photographs of his profile used for scientific purposes, but not those of his full face. "I may bump into some doctor who has seen my pictures. I want to forget all this and not have others know. It's not that I'm ashamed of what I've done, but I just want to forget it." Eleven months later he was still convinced of the wisdom of his decision to alter his appearance.

It was the best thing that ever happened to me. My whole life is changed. I feel like a human being. If I were to write a book, I'd call it "Knock on Any Door," because that is what I can do now. Every day I have another reason for being glad I changed my nose. When I'm introduced to people I feel I create an interest, particularly with women. They look at me with more interest and intentness. I can go in any group and be accepted. As a rule, a Jew becomes uncomfortable in the presence of a Gentile, especially if he doesn't want to show it—the way I did.

Arthur said it no longer made any difference to him if an individual were a Gentile or a Jew. He was living at home, and his friends in the neighborhood were Jewish. "I can afford to be generous and accept Jews now because I know I don't look like one. Before, I identified myself with them and resisted them." On occasion he had "tested" his belief that he no longer appeared Jewish by making remarks in Yiddish to salesmen in Jewish shops. "They won't bite. They think I'm trying to be smart. They don't know I'm a Jew."

Arthur felt that he had "built up a personality" with his "new face and name," but he wanted "one more thing," on which he was working at the time of our final interview—to rid himself of speech characteristics that he thought identified him with a specific urban area. "Good speech is a product of your environment, and, if you want to get into good circles, you must sound like the cultured people in them. I want to be more than just an ordinary guy now."

YOU OUGHT TO BE ABLE TO LIE IN THE SUN.

The Case of David Stein

David Stein, age 18, was accompanied by his mother when he came to the surgeon's office to request a rhinoplasty. His was a very prominent nose, not unduly long but had a high nasal hump. His other facial features were good. He had blond hair, blue eyes, and somewhat resembled Danny Kaye. Both he and Mrs. Stein were attractively dressed.

David had an alert mind but appeared irritable and disconsolate. During the interview he slumped in his chair, was on the defensive, and was openly hostile toward his mother, who frequently interrupted or prodded him to "tell the truth." He said he had no breathing difficulties; he just wanted his nose "changed."

> I first became conscious of my nose when I matured—and when I became aware of it socially. Others made remarks about it. I used to take it seriously, but realized I couldn't hide myself. It has caused me a lot of anguish. I could be so much more self-confident if it were changed. My other features are good—it's just this one thing. Many times I have been inhibited—like meeting new people. I would hesitate going places and sometimes didn't go.

David and his family were Conservative Jews. Mrs. Stein attended Temple regularly, and all members of the family observed the High Holy Days. David was also a member of the Society for the Advancement of Judaism. Mr. Stein, American-born of Russian parents, was a successful salesman in a clothing firm. His Russian-born wife was an ambitious and dominating woman who rationalized her overprotectiveness and her strictness with David as "wanting to do the right thing by him." He, on the other hand, felt that his life had been "too sheltered and protected." He resented the fact that his mother was "always making me feel guilty about things that are perfectly normal. She criticizes my friends, and she won't let me go anywhere—not even out of the city to work during Christmas vacation. That's why I want to go West to college so that I can get away from her influence."

David had two brothers: one 25 and married, the other 14. Both had straight and shapely noses like their mother's. David resented not only the fact that his nose was different—"Why did I have to be the only one in the family to get this nose?"—but also that his older brother was the "favorite" child—"My father was always talking about the big plans he had for him. Then, when my younger brother arrived, *he* was the baby and the favorite."

Whereas David's brothers, according to Mrs. Stein, were "very smart in school, models of behavior, and never caused us any trouble," David was "the problem." He did poorly in school because he "didn't apply himself." He was mischievous and had been caught smoking. A few weeks before high school graduation he failed in chemistry. The teacher was "one of those New Englanders"; in David's opinion, he was domineering and ridiculed the students—"I was the only one who saw his shortcomings, and I blew up one day." David was dismissed from the class and subsequently failed in the course, which prevented his graduating. While waiting to enroll for the next term he had gone to work in his father's firm. He also had enrolled in an evening art class. But a month later he had been forced to give up his class and to curtail his daily working hours because of what Mrs. Stein described as a slight "physical and mental breakdown," due to overwork.

According to David and his mother, religious discrimination did not enter into his desire to change his nose. "Having my nose changed," he said, "won't make me lose my Jewishness. It's just that a person who doesn't have a prominent nose wouldn't think twice about doing things that one who has one does." To corroborate his point, Mrs. Stein interrupted to tell of a Jewish boy they knew who had "a good nose" but whose name caused him trouble. "When he changed it from Leibowitz to Lee, I said, 'Maybe so, but you're still Leibowitz to me.'"

Mr. Stein, she continued, had a nose "identical to David's, and three years ago he had it changed."

But it was not due to discrimination. All our friends are Jewish. He travels a lot, and even in the South—where he has non-Jewish friends—he has never come across any discrimination. He wasn't self-conscious about his nose the way David is. After all, he is much older and married. But he said he felt that the boys were getting older and soon would be getting married, and he'd have to meet prospective daughter-in-laws [sic] and their relatives, and he thought he'd look better if his nose was changed. Also, his niece had hers changed, and he said if she could do it, so could he. These were the reasons he gave.

Then, as if to justify her husband's action, Mrs. Stein added, "In fact, at our Temple recently a Jewish psychiatrist said, 'If Jews hate their noses, they should get them changed.'" David interjected:

> The thing is that plastic surgery has become so prominent lately that I decided six months ago to have it done. I'm doing most of the things I want to do, but I just feel I will be more confident in doing them than I am now. I have a charming personality, and that makes up for a lot, but in business my nose would be a handicap. The ability is there, but ability is not enough.

"Both his brothers have good noses," said Mrs. Stein, "and sometimes his older brother makes remarks about David's nose" —"So do *you*," David retorted, adding bitterly, "Even at home remarks are made."

When he traveled on buses and subways people stared at his nose, David said, and made him so self-conscious that he resorted to such devices as keeping his head turned to prevent his profile from being seen. He never wore a hat because he felt it would make his nose more conspicuous. "Why do I have to go through all these contortions because of my nose?" he asked.

David said he was unable to remember any specific incidents or remarks about his nose. "I can't recall remarks or my feelings about them back more than two years. Maybe I want to repress them. I get madder at myself than at those who make remarks. *They* are stupid—*I'm* not—and it makes me angry at myself for feeling this way." In high school, he claimed, he had never met with any discrimination. "Most students in school were Jewish. If I had met it [discrimination] I'd be worse off than I am now. But, I'd just as soon not advertise my Jewishness and would be just as glad if people aren't sure whether I'm Jewish or not. I'd rather have them know me as an individual first."

David's lack of sociability in school had troubled both his mother and the principal. Although he had occasionally gone to dances or had weekend dates, he showed little interest in girls. "I can take them or leave them," he said arrogantly. "They don't constitute [sic] any of my time. I get around fairly well." As for the other boys in school, "They were just not my type." The subject of friends precipitated a heated argument between David and Mrs. Stein. "I have one real friend," he said bitterly, "and she doesn't approve of him." (This was 18-year-old

Harold, who was Jewish.) "No," his mother explained, "Harold has bad manners. I don't like his political affiliations, and I'm afraid he will influence David." "It's because he's poor that you don't like him," remonstrated David. "Maybe he doesn't have good manners, but he's more intelligent than any other boy I know—he's so far above the average." Then he added, "I choose friends who have inferiority complexes too, because then I don't have to feel inferior and can even feel superior to them. This boy has a large nose, too. We discuss our noses and commiserate with each other."

Although David's operation had been routine, Mrs. Stein was visibly anxious about it and overly upset when he developed a slight hemorrhage. A week after surgery the dressing was removed. David was both startled and immensely pleased by the result. Beaming, he entered the adjoining room where his mother waited. (She had refused to watch while the dressing was removed.) At first glance she gasped, "Oh! David!" and covered her face with her hands. "It's a wonderful job, but I can't get used to it. I don't know my own son!" Holding out her hands to him she said, "Let's get acquainted again!" David kept smiling, looking in the mirror, and asking, "Do you like it, Mom?"

Alone with the interviewer David revealed the deep bitterness and conflict of his feelings, which a change in appearance had not removed. "I like my new nose, but I'm angry because it must be changed. Why must we *have* to say what kind of noses we want in this world? I don't think noses should have to be changed, yet I did it." He described again how self-conscious he had been, adding that the trouble he had in school and his poor personal relations might have been caused by resentment about his nose, "discrimination, and maybe other things too."

A week later David returned to the office, this time by himself. He was obviously less tense and was anxious to talk. He no longer slumped in his chair nor looked sullen, as he had in his mother's presence at the first interview. He looked happy and repeatedly stated how delighted he was with the surgical results, saying that the first thing he had done was to go out and buy a hat. He described with pleasure the "shock" his father had when he saw him. "He was so pleased at the change! He said I look like an Irishman now! My friends say I look terrific, and the girls at work call me a 'handsome-looking guy.' I feel good."

David described the sense of freedom he experienced in subways and other public places. "Not to be worrying if people are looking at your profile is a relief. It gives you a wonderful sense of security because you know your nose is good, and you can concentrate on other things. I would have been a neurotic if this wasn't done. Not until we talked here in the office that first day did my mother realize how much this had concerned me. It cleared a lot of things between us, such as her overprotectiveness and my friendship with Harold."

Harold, David thought, was feeling "a certain discomfort" with him "because my nose is changed. He seems to have respect for me though. He is the only one who can really appreciate why I had it done. And I did it," David blurted out, "purely because of discrimination." Self-consciousness about the shape of his nose and its social significance had begun in junior high school, he said, when he was about 13. An Italian boy had made a remark about David's religion, and a fight ensued. At that time he was living in a Jewish neighborhood bordered by Irish and Italians.

> If I were out walking with a girl or other Jewish boys, the Irish and Italian kids would gang around and make cracks or deliberately incite riots. It got too dangerous to walk along the parkway. . . . If I lived in a Utopia I wouldn't have to change my nose. There wouldn't be any discrimination because of religion or the shape of a nose. I'm resentful now of society. We shouldn't be made to feel different and out of things.

David's dislike and resentment of his nose and his preoccupation with it had grown to such an extent that for the past two years he had left open a mirrored closet door near his bed so that he would not see his face the last thing at night and the first thing in the morning. "The night I went home with my new nose," he said, "I closed that door. It's been closed ever since. *Now* I can look at myself."

A month later David appeared voluntarily at the office and wanted to talk about his friend, Harold, who was unhappy and "worried about his nose." David wanted to help him have a rhinoplasty. Harold could not afford an operation, but David and another friend planned to pool their savings and pay for it. He knew Harold wanted surgery because of the things he said and did.

Now that my nose is fixed, he'll look at me and say, "Gee, you're a handsome ape!" The other day we were lying on the grass in the park. I felt so at ease and was sprawled out with my face to the sun and toward the people walking by. Harold kept the back of his head toward everyone. He couldn't get any sun. He knew I knew why he lay in that position. He can't go through life like that. You ought to be able to lie in the sun. I know how it feels. He knows he can't afford an operation and has tried to adjust himself, but he sees that I've had mine done, and it makes it harder for him. When I suggested he have an operation he cried, because he knew I realized how much he was suffering. He feels society should be corrected, but he can't go off to Mars. He's felt more discrimination than I have. He's been less sheltered and around more. It's [race prejudice] in his neighborhood, and he's been subjected to more. His family are from the Old Country and don't understand what these things are all about.

Harold is aggressive and unconventional in his behavior. He is neurotic already, and I'm afraid it will become worse on account of his nose. He is extremely intelligent, but in social affairs with a nose like that he has to settle for a beast [second best]. Otherwise he could have the most beautiful girl. He makes fun of himself. He has a fast technique with the girls so they don't notice his nose. He'll say "I've got beautiful blond hair—a perfect physique —what if my nose *is* long?" He's acting. It will catch up with him —all this compensation. You can't do it indefinitely. I know what it's like.

Even I have developed a superior feeling and can talk more about others' noses. I can afford to joke about them, though even noticing a person with a big nose is wrong. After my operation my mother compared Harold's nose to Jimmy Durante's. She said, "He's the black sheep around here now. *We* all have *good* noses." She can make cracks now because we all have good noses. Before, it would have hurt me—with my nose—yet it hurts anyway, because of Harold.

However, there were more pleasant things resulting from his operation that David wanted to report. When he returned to work, his superior did not recognize him. "He was so impressed he said he wished he could have *his* nose changed!" In a clothing store where David had accompanied Harold, the salesman said to the latter, "If you were as handsome as your brother here, you wouldn't have any trouble finding clothes." "This never happened before," David said, "this kind of comparison. Before it was always the reverse."

One of the most spectacular results of his changed appearance was the manner in which his father had reacted.

> He keeps looking at me. He's more thrilled than I am. Now he goes out of his way to introduce me to his customers, and he wants to take me on a trip with him. This never happened before. In our business, impressions are important. Before, everything depended on my appearance, and my nose was against me. In a way it's really pitiful. Father wasn't ashamed of me before, exactly, but now he wants me along. He's more relaxed with me. I can sense it walking down the street with him. Before his nose was fixed he wasn't self-conscious about me, but after his operation there was a certain distance between us. Now he's proud of me.

In these two cases there are basic personality problems and emotional disturbances that have their roots in early childhood and in family relationships. The focus here, however, is on some of the salient sociopsychological and cultural determinants in the responses of two young men to their ethnic visibility.

Arthur's obvious neurosis is centered around two conflicts, both of which involve important cultural values. One is related to the fact that his is not a typical Jewish family. His father's excessive drinking and abuse of his wife, behavior contrary to Jewish cultural patterns, cause him shame and unhappiness. As a child he makes few friends; as an adult he seeks acceptance by Gentiles, whom he tends to identify as Irish. The second conflict is the discrepancy between his strong intellectual ambitions, consistent with Jewish values, and his scanty education.

Frustrated in his desire to be accepted and successful, Arthur makes use of the stereotype to explain his difficulties, employing his Jewishness as a pivotal point. First, he changes his name. Then he decides to alter the shape of his nose. He claims that his inability to make friends and to achieve success is due to his "Jewish" nose. Because of it he can not have a part in a play. Since his nose indicates his ethnic origin, he cannot attract Gentile friends. Manifestations of anti-Semitism in the army increased his sensitivity to his Jewishness and presumably accelerated his desire to pass among Gentiles as a non-Jew.

Though Arthur has encountered anti-Semitism, at no time is he able to cope overtly with the reality of prejudice and discrimination. Although his inner reactions are violent, he remains outwardly passive: "Jews don't fight." Anyway, it is the "lower-level people" he blames. Despite the immediate and apparent candor of his initial statement that discrimination is his problem, he constructs elaborate rationalizations for requesting rhinoplasty. He says he wants to advance himself and associate with superior intellectual people, not to pass as a Gentile—just to "have the subject [Jewishness] dropped" and to "stop running."

At the same time he fears that surgery will cut him off from his family, particularly his mother. (Note his later statement: "The umbilical cord has been cut"). She says: "It's going to hurt you, and if it hurts you it will hurt me."[30] "God gave it to you" (the traditional Jewish attitude toward mutilation). But, to justify what might appear to other Jews to be a renunciation of his faith and to assuage his guilt feelings about changing his identity, he will become a catalyst, a "good-will ambassador" to prove to Gentiles that he is "not only a 'white man' but a 'white Jew.'" (His stereotypes of Jews are couched in Gentile terms.)

Postoperatively his basic and deep attachment to his Jewish origin is expressed in the shock he receives when he sees himself. "I was horrified when I looked like an Irishman. I was a man without a country. . . . A Jew has tremendous pride. . . . I didn't want to lose the link with something I was most accustomed to."

When the "rational" and visible obstacle to making friends and being a success had been removed, and his relations with other Jews and with his mother are not severed (she says he looks "wonderful"), he feels free and happy. "I think I'd prefer to marry a Jewish girl. We'd understand each other better." "I'd like to be a philosopher—the kind of philosophic Jew—quiet and wise."

[30] For a psychocultural analysis of this rather common response of Jewish mothers see Wolfenstein, Martha, "Two Types of Jewish Mothers" in *Childhood in Contemporary Cultures*, edited by Margaret Mead and Martha Wolfenstein. University of Chicago Press, Chicago, 1955, pp. 424–440.

(Although the dedicated learned man is a Jewish cultural ideal, again it is Arthur's own stereotype that is revealed.)

Nevertheless, Arthur remains ambivalent. He can neither wholly embrace his own people nor relinquish them.[31] He wants Jews to know he's a Jew, but not Gentiles. Nor has he "stopped running." He wishes to rid himself of speech mannerisms he considers socially handicapping. He wants to be "more than just an ordinary guy."

In contrast to Arthur, David at first states unequivocally that discrimination does not enter into his wish for a rhinoplasty. He wants it, he claims, because he is "the only one in the family" with such a prominent nose, and it makes him self-conscious. As if to lend credence to David's rationale, his mother cites her husband's reason for having his nose changed: namely, to "look better," as his sons are getting older and he will be meeting prospective daughters-in-law. To support the legitimacy of having a rhinoplasty she quotes the Jewish psychiatrist's approving dictum. Although David himself disclaims experiencing religious prejudice or discrimination, he indicates concern about his visibility as a Jew.

Postoperatively, David's newfound sense of security allows him to make a more realistic appraisal of his reasons for wanting his nose changed. He recalls incidents of his earlier life that he had formerly suppressed, and expresses his fear of discrimination and his deep resentment of society. At the same time, removal of his handicap has reduced personal and family tensions and has strengthened his self-concept. His former self-preoccupation is replaced by his empathy with and compassion for his friend, Harold, with whom he still identifies himself.

These two cases demonstrate the attempt to fuse a number of conflicting attitudes and feelings into a solution of their problems

[31] For discussion of similar conflicts experienced by partly assimilated Jews, see Wirth, Louis, *The Ghetto*, University of Chicago Press, Chicago, 1928, pp. 263–281.

by having rhinoplasty. Both patients were concerned about their noses as clues to their ethnic identity and as stimuli to negative reactions. The degree to which their responses were functions of reality, however, differed.

Arthur's response was far out of proportion to the reality of his situation. Threatened by his group identification, he sought to change it. Not only did he use what he conceived to be the dominant Jewish stereotype as the source of his frustration, but he deprecated characteristics he identified as Jewish and in doing so manifested what Kurt Lewin called "negative chauvinism."[32] Surgery effected cosmetic change, but, because Arthur lacked insight into his real problems, psychological results were superficial. Still unable to accept himself, he remained in social and psychological limbo. David's response, on the other hand, was in greater degree realistic, and for him surgery had a therapeutic effect.

Irrespective of the reality or nonreality of these two patients' complaints, as well as those of the other Jewish patients interviewed, they are reflections of the role played by perceptual factors in human relations. Where the social stereotypes of a group are discrediting, a person threatened by his identification with it may seek to conceal his membership in it. Changing the shape of his nose is an expression of the wish to reduce his ethnic visibility and to have his appearance conform to that of the favored majority. In doing so, however, his self-evaluation may reflect not only his inability to accept himself but also negative attributes that he imputes to his group.

Whether or not the felt need for surgery is symptomatic of psychological disturbance or a deep-seated neurosis—and there is substantial evidence that such conditions are common among rhinoplasty patients[33]—the socially and culturally defined attitudes and prejudices toward persons of certain ethnic back-

[32] Lewin, Kurt, *Resolving Social Conflicts*, edited by Gertrud W. Lewin, Harper and Bros., New York, 1948, p. 193.

[33] Linn, Louis and Irving B. Goldman, "Psychiatric Observations Concerning Rhinoplasty," op. cit., pp. 307-314; also, Macgregor, Frances Cooke and Bertram Schaffner, op. cit., pp. 277-291.

grounds provide strong impetus for seeking rhinoplasty. In other words, regarding the nose as an impediment is not necessarily or solely the manifestation of a neurotic personality, but the expression of a sociopsychological and cultural phenomenon.

CHAPTER FIVE

Congenital Anomaly:
The Malformed Child
and the Family

THE COMPLEX OF PROBLEMS

I have a baby born with a birthmark on the right side of her face and head. It extends out from the corner of her eye down to her neck and chest and back over her ear and into the back of her head, quite a large area. It is quite red but not raised. I know it cannot be removed, but that is not the problem. The problem is that I am at a loss as to how to answer all the people who tell me how terrible it looks and ask why I don't do something about it. I have tried staying away from those people but, needless to say, that is not easy to do. We live in a small town and already there are two stores I don't patronize any more as the clerks told me her face looks terrible. So I am wondering if you have pamphlets that would answer some of the questions that need to be answered both to me and all the ignorant people in this small town of ours. She has a twin sister who does not have a mark. I don't want her to grow up with any emotional problem resulting from this. So any information you can send me regarding this condition will be greatly appreciated.   (a mother)

The stigmata of congenital facial anomalies present a special order of problems. Since few such defects can be corrected in infancy, whereas others may require multiple surgical procedures, the fitting of prostheses, and intermittent hospitalizations over a period of years, they create a variety of social, psychological, and economic stresses that impinge upon and endanger the emotional and mental equilibrium of both the child and the family.

Compounding these difficulties are the prevailing prejudices and beliefs with respect to cause and effect. More than one might suppose in this scientifically enlightened age, superstitions about the causes of congenital deformities persist. It has been documented in our interviews with patients that many people attribute certain types of anomalies to the mother's experiences during pregnancy: A harelip, for example, to her having touched a rabbit or suffered severe fright or seen an eclipse of the moon. But more commonly a child's deformity is interpreted as God's punishment for some transgression or negligence on the part of the parents. And it has been noted that even medically knowledgeable people who say they realize it is not "scientifically sound" are frequently nagged by the notion that somehow the parents are responsible for the misfortune.

Not uncommon, either, is the assumption that the physically defective child is likely to be mentally retarded as well, an affliction that calls up strong social and emotional associations. Indeed, cases are known of malformed children being mistakenly placed in institutions for the mentally retarded. Treated *as if* they were retarded, they became socially retarded, which in turn falsely validates the original assumption. Even doctors may unquestioningly accept the association of mental deficiency with congenital malformation. A 7-year-old girl, during several visits to a plastic surgery clinic for evaluation of her gross facial deformity and partial deafness, was assumed to be mentally retarded. A medical report from the referring physician had included the statement: "This patient also has dental problems," but in his rapid reading the resident-surgeon, after he had seen the child, saw the word as "mental." It came as a shock to the staff to learn that the child was exceptionally bright.

PARENTAL ATTITUDES AND BEHAVIOR*

Because of society's attitude toward those whose faces deviate from the norm, a universal reaction to giving birth to a facially deformed infant is one of dismay, with varying degrees of shock, grief, anger, or shame. Following the first shock of learning that her baby has a facial defect are the mother's inevitable questions: What did I do to deserve this? Why did this have to happen to me? What was the cause? Was it my fault? The father's?

* See Notes at back of book.

Sometimes when a child is born with a deformity the doctors and nurses delay telling the mother. But silence and mystery surrounding such events may be more harrowing than reality.[1] A woman whose child was born with a defective ear put it this way:

Nobody told me anything. They just didn't bring the baby in to me, and this made me apprehensive. Eventually a student nurse, in response to my questions, blurted out that the baby was "deformed in some way." I had visions of something with hooves and really made a scene until everyone came running and finally produced little Tommy, at which time I immediately calmed down.

From the time a child with a facial abnormality is born, the obstetrician, pediatrician, and nurse are in strategic positions to aid the parents by dispelling the myths about retribution and "maternal impressions," by explaining the nature and cause, if known, of the defect and by giving information and reassurance about the possibilities of surgical treatment. It comforts the parents to learn that a cleft lip, for example, may be operable within weeks or months, in which case the psychological effects on the child will be negligible. In other types of anomalies, however, surgical intervention may have to be delayed until cranial and facial bones have grown larger.

Parental attitudes and behavior toward a child with a congenital facial anomaly are of critical importance to the adaptation and adjustment he will make as he grows up. If the parents feel shame, resentment, or guilt, these feelings can be conveyed even to an infant, for an infant is responsive to the tenseness of his mother's body. Some parents, to allay a lurking sense of guilt or to compensate for his handicap, become overprotective and indulgent, giving him more attention than they give their other children. Conversely, some parents openly reject the anomalous

[1] In his study of the impact of giving birth to children with cleft lip and palate, Clifford found that the longer the delay in telling the mother and showing her child to her, the greater the "expressed impact." Clifford, Edward, "Cleft Palate and the Person: Psychological Studies of Its Impact," *Journal of the Southern Medical Association*, vol. 64, no. 12, 1971, pp. 1516–1520.

child and favor his siblings. In both instances the child feels different and set apart, and thus the way is paved for emotional and behavioral disorders.[2]

While there are no simple solutions to the problems that are bound to confront the family of a congenitally deformed child, the following cases demonstrate that early professional and continued guidance can make the difference between eventual adjustment and irreversible psychic damage:

When Mrs. S. saw newborn Nathan's face she became hysterical. What should have been his right ear was a small fleshy nodule on the lower side of his cheek, the side of his face was lopsided, the right eye abnormal in shape, and his tiny receding chin deviated to one side. During the first few months of Nathan's life no one outside the family was allowed to see him. When friends finally visited, Mrs. S. held Nathan's defective side against her body. When taking him out for an airing she covered his head with a frilled bonnet to conceal his deformity. Sensing her parents' shame his 6-year-old sister hid him in a corner when her friends came to play.

At 2½ years of age Nathan was brought by his mother from their home in Israel to New York for plastic surgery. His behavior already reflected the family's attitudes and extreme anxiety. He screamed when his hat was removed and hid his face in his mother's skirts. Weeping, Mrs. S. reported: "I think he's already developed an inferiority complex. Even in the house he runs to put his hat on if anyone comes, or hides in another room."

The surgeons, as had her doctor in Israel, told Mrs. S. that surgery would be inadvisable until Nathan was in his teens. Meanwhile Mrs. S. was strongly urged to cut her son's hair

[2] For a detailed discussion of parents' attitudes toward and management of their children with deformities, see: Lauer, Edith, "The Family," and Bryt, Albert, "Psychiatric Aspects," in *Facial Deformities and Plastic Surgery: A Psychosocial Study*, Macgregor, et al., Charles C Thomas, Springfield, Illinois, 1953, pp. 103-129.

[3] This took place before long hair on boys was acceptable.

(which she had kept long to hide his ear),[3] to discard his cap, to stop overprotecting him, and to allow him the same freedom of movement as his sister. In view of her own agitated state it was suggested that Mrs. S. have psychiatric help. These suggestions she temporarily accepted, but later disregarded them when greatly disappointed she returned to her home.

In a letter from her a year later she reported that her husband, who interpreted having an imperfect son as a reflection on his masculinity, was very angry because she had brought the child home instead of leaving him with relatives in New York until he could have surgery. "He is ashamed of the boy." Her daughter, who had been told her brother would come home with a "new face," was so upset by his appearance that "to have any peace in the family," she had been sent to camp, a financial burden her parents could ill afford. At age 4, Nathan, who was a bright child, was placed in kindergarten, but the taunts of other children sent him home in tears "crying for two ears like the others have." In desperation Mrs. S. took Nathan to a doctor whose several attempts to construct an ear actually worsened his appearance.

By the age of 8 Nathan was seriously maladjusted and unmanageable. On one occasion, for instance, his mother came home to find him hysterical. He had been looking in the mirror and was "breaking up everything around the house." Turning on her he said: "You had no right to let me live when I look like this. What's going to happen to me later?" Shortly thereafter when some boys at school tore off the dressing his parents made him wear and called him "monster," he went down to the beach and tried to drown himself. On another occasion he tried to asphyxiate himself in the kitchen and when revived cried because they wouldn't "let him go."

When Nathan was 12 his mother, now "too nervous" to leave home, sent him to New York to live with relatives while, as they hoped, reconstructive surgery could be started. When seen at the clinic he was depressed and withdrawn. He was still wearing a dressing. Psychological tests indicated that while he appeared to have average intellectual potentiality, his performance was hampered by anxieties and preoccupations. The projective test findings indicated an isolation of self in a world lacking warmth and acceptance.

> He feels like a wounded animal, different, isolated, and rejected. Since no one likes him he ends up hating himself and the world. He is afraid to act out his hostility because he expects that lowering his guard will expose him to worse things that could happen to him. His relationship with the father figure is inadequate for the development of masculine identity, and he is extremely ambivalent about the mother figure which he views as cold and aggressive. There is a possibility that failure of his hopes from surgery may plunge him into depression and there may be a recurrence of suicidal attempts.

An operation to correct Nathan's eye was first performed with satisfactory results. It was decided, however, that both jaw surgery and attempts to construct an ear should be delayed since scar tissue from the earlier ear operations made a successful outcome extremely dubious and, considering Nathan's precarious psychological state, it was feared that an ear operation at this time might entail serious risk. Moreover, because jaw surgery could interfere with the growth process, the surgeon recommended that this too be deferred until Nathan was older. He did suggest, however, that to make Nathan more comfortable with himself and others he be fitted with a prosthetic ear. But neither this suggestion nor the earlier recommendations of psychiatric help or counselling for both the boy and his mother were accepted. Again, Nathan returned home.

At age 19 Nathan went to live in a kibbutz; his deformity prevented his acceptance into the army. In the kibbutz he went to school, learned to farm and to repair tractors. He also received some surgical attention.

At our last report Nathan, now 25, was still in the kibbutz and working as a mechanic. He wears a prosthetic ear and has had some corrective surgery of his jaw. To his family's dismay, he refuses to consider any job on the outside for which he might be paid and says he plans to live in the kibbutz the rest of his life.

In contrast is the experience of Mr. and Mrs. P. and their daughter Rachel, who was born with a pigmented hairy nevus that covered the entire right side of her face. Distraught, they sought the help of a plastic surgeon when she was 8 months old and, being highly receptive to psychological counselling, they conscientiously followed the suggestion to rear her as nearly as possible as they would a nondisfigured child.

As might be expected, they went through times of deep despair. Surgery had to be carried out in stages, with periods when improvement was hard to see. Within twenty-two years, 34 operations were performed. Anxiety and worry were compounded by financial strain and a developing tension between the parents. But all this time the counselor maintained contact with the family, and during critical phases the help of psychiatrists was enlisted. Rachel still carries visible scars, but she has suffered no serious psychological damage. She is outgoing, has considerable charm, and is now happily married.

CONSCIOUSNESS OF DIFFERENCE

The onset of "stigma learning" may be gradual or sudden, but sooner or later it is bound to occur.[4] A child of preschool age may well realize that he has a port-wine stain or only one eye, yet remain untroubled by it. Sustained by accepting and loving parents, protected in a warm, accepting environment, he is spared, during the critical years at least, knowledge of the social implications and consequences of being different. Other children, however, may be less fortunate. Because a child is too young to talk or to express his feelings in words, adults tend to assume that he is unaware that "something is wrong." Overlooked, however, are the sensory responses of an infant to its mother's kinesthetic behavior: As already indicated, if she is anxious, fearful or angry, her feelings may be communicated to the child who, in turn, senses that something is amiss.

[4] Goffman, Erving, *Stigma: Notes on the Management of Spoiled Identity*. Prentice-Hall, Englewood Cliffs, New Jersey, 1963, p. 33.

Even before the child can talk he may notice something different about his own face. One mother reported seeing her 18-month-old daughter who, catching sight of herself in a mirror, immediately rubbed her finger over her markedly malformed nose. Kresky and Simon cite the case of a boy born with a hairy nevus that covered half his face:

> From the age of 18 months the patient spent a great deal of time looking out the window at a small white dog with a large brown patch on his face. Occasionally he would leave the window and cry bitterly. As he began to talk, he showed confusion in identity, frequently referring to the dog as "baby" and to himself as "bow-wow." He repeated "bow-wow, boo-boo," "Who has the boo-boo?" (pointing to birthmark). "Where does baby have boo-boo?" (pointing to the dog). On one occasion the patient saw an infant in a carriage, put his hand up to his face, touched the nevus, pointed to the baby and screamed, "Baby, baby, no boo-boo. Where is boo-boo?"[5]

At 19 months the patient had already undergone two of a series of procedures for removal of the nevus. A third operation, however, was a tonsillectomy. When he subsequently saw himself in the mirror, he pointed to his right cheek and burst into sobs. That night he had an attack of colic, vomiting, and diarrhea, the first of several somatic expressions of his anxiety about his appearance.

Though little children may be puzzled or hurt by the reactions of others, they are especially vulnerable to being found deficient in the eyes of their mothers and fathers. Erik Erikson writes of young childhood as a critical time in the formation of identity: Speaking of the child at the age of 3 he says, "Being firmly convinced that he is a person on his own, the child must now find out what kind of person he may become. . . ."[6] Former plastic surgery patients seen in the course of a 20-year follow-up study[7] have reported that discrediting remarks, unwittingly made by a parent had, initially or in retrospect, triggered or intensified feelings of differentness and inadequacy.

[5] Kresky, Beatrice, and Bernard E. Simon, "Infantile Reaction to Facial Disfigurement," *Archives of Surgery*, vol. 82, May 1961, pp. 783–788.

[6] Erikson, Erik H., *Identity, Youth, and Crisis*, W. W. Norton, New York, 1968, p. 115.

[7] This study by the writer is currently under way at New York University Medical Center, Institute of Reconstructive Plastic Surgery.

Such, for example, was the experience of two 7-year-old boys, each of whom had a partially missing ear and was in the interoperative stage of surgical reconstruction. Wide-eyed and immobile, they sat in the clinic room with their mothers, looking from one woman to another absorbed in their conversation.

Mrs. A: What makes me angry is the adults. Children I don't mind so much, as they are naturally curious. But when grown-up people come up and ask me "What's the matter with your little boy?" it makes me angry. You'd think they would have more sense. When I tell them sometimes they react with horror.

Mrs. B: A woman came up to me not long ago and said, "I've seen all your children, and I've never asked you about Jeffrey, but I've wondered if I could ask you a question," and I said, "You want to know about his ear," and she said, "Yes." I told her it was a birth defect and that he was having surgery for it and it would be fixed. This seemed to satisfy her.

Mrs. A: Well, you knew the woman and she was interested. It's when people are total strangers that it makes you mad when they ask you questions.

Both women had had children following the birth of their afflicted sons, and they discussed their trepidation about additional pregnancies.

Mrs. A: You know you can't help wondering if it's going to happen again and there will be something wrong with the next one. When the new baby came, I wanted to know right away if everything was where it was supposed to be.

Mrs. B: Yes, that's what I was worried about, too. I told them to look at the baby and tell me if everything was all right. I didn't want to find out that there was anything wrong with her.

Some parents, deluded into thinking that if neither they nor the child mention his deformity he will not be disturbed by it, shun the subject and behave as if it did not exist. Such avoidance, however, may lead him to assume that his defect is a tabooed topic and in some way "bad," which may, as the following case illustrates, only increase his sensitiveness.

Ten-year-old Bobby was good looking except for conspicuous lop ears. He never referred to them, nor did his parents, who took it for granted that his appearance did not worry him. They believed he would not take an interest in his looks until he reached puberty, at which time, if he wished, he could have an operation. For two years they had been concerned about "more serious" problems. Bobby was troubled by enuresis,[8] which continued despite medical treatment. At school the teacher complained that he failed to concentrate, cried easily, was sometimes incontinent, and, although he was bright, his grades had fallen below average. Both in and out of school he sought children much younger than himself, assiduously avoiding his peers. Distressing to his mother was the discovery that he had pilfered money from her purse to buy candy for his playmates. It had not occurred to his parents, doctors, or teachers that there might be a relationship between his lop ears and his behavior. This possibility did, however, enter the mind of a new teacher, who noticed other children teasing him, and suggested plastic surgery to his mother.

Bobby was delighted at the prospect of having his ears corrected and during a preoperative interview told why. For a long time, he said, other children had made fun of him. They had nicknamed him "Donkey Ears," and "Dumbo," and had told him that he "looked like a taxicab going around the corner with both doors open." Feeling powerless to cope with boys his own age, he took refuge among younger children seeking their approval by giving them candy.

A month after surgery, Bobby's mother reported that his enuresis had ceased and that both his school work and his behavior had shown marked improvement.

THE CASE OF FRANCISCO RODRIGUEZ

The expanded case history that follows is intended to illustrate in greater detail two aspects of the plight of the child with a malformed face and his family, how the prevailing mores in the

---

[8] Incontinence of urine.

world around them enter into the common interpretations of facial deformities, and how, in the intimate world of the family, these interpretations may in turn determine the whole network of personal relationships.

Francisco was an 8-year-old Venezuelan boy who was born without a left ear. In place of an external auditory canal were two small vestigial remains of auricular cartilage. Further down the cheek and out of normal position was a small lobule.

Attractive, well-developed, and large for his age, Francisco was aggressive, mentally alert, and extremely active. In striking contrast to his manly build and demeanor, however, was his long bobbed hair (not fashionable at the time), which served to conceal his deformity and made him look like a cross between Tom Sawyer and Little Lord Fauntleroy. His family, who had brought him to New York for surgical construction of the ear, included his father, a tall, good-looking man to whom he was obviously attached and whom he kissed on the slightest pretext; his mother, a quiet, retiring woman; and his 10-year-old sister. Although they all watched over him with marked protectiveness, he seemed indifferent to their concern and constant attention.

Francisco's father, a dentist, was highly emotional about his son's deformity, and his voice quavered when he described the anxiety and suffering it had caused him and his wife. For eight years they had planned and waited for the day when the boy could have plastic surgery. The trip to New York had involved great personal and financial sacrifice, yet Mr. Rodriguez said repeatedly that no sacrifice was too great if Francisco could be made to look normal. Both parents were eager to donate cartilage from their ears to make one for their son, and they were both disappointed and alarmed to learn that cartilage would be taken from his own rib.

Dr. Rodriguez had realized the difficulty: ". . . a constructed ear may look misshapen, but people will probably assume it was caused by an accident, which is not as bad as having a birth defect. With no ear the boy could never have a happy life." He explained that Francisco's hair had been kept long to cover his "orejita mala" ("bad little ear;" always so referred to and never as a defect or deformity). In this way they had "prevented him from developing a complex about it, because others would not notice it and make derogatory remarks." The boy therefore "never worries about his ear, and he never speaks of it because he has been forbidden to do so. But he is a big boy now and he hates having his hair long. He is always asking to have it cut so he will look like other boys or like me."

Dr. Rodriguez and his family are people of moderate means. They live in Caracas where the doctor is well-known in his community and respected in his profession. While he is very fond of his wife, whom he regards as a "child," and of his daughter Clara, his son is the main object of his affection and attention.

Prior to Francisco's birth, the Rodriguez couple participated in the customary social activities of their group: frequent Sunday and holiday picnics with other families. They took part in the fiestas, belonged to the tennis club, and engaged in a great deal of visiting with friends and relatives. Although they were not particularly devout Catholics, they attended church with fair regularity.

When Francisco was born, his deformity was "a great shock and disappointment." His parents feared his defect would "always be an object of curiosity" and a source of "shame and humiliation . . . for them all." Furthermore, he might be "marked" by the handicap. Dr. Rodriguez remembered the professor he had in school who was born without an ear; how he and the other boys referred to him as "One Ear" and made fun of him. Although considered successful in his work, the professor's life was marred by his deformity—"He lived an abnormal life; he never married nor participated in social activities of any kind, and he finally became a recluse." But Dr. Rodriguez would not allow his son to be subjected to the ridicule of other children, or to deprecatory nicknames; he did not want him to develop "complexes about his bad little ear," or to be ashamed or timid because he was "different."

Within a month of Francisco's birth, his parents decided that he should be isolated as much as possible and his defect concealed to avoid "embarrassing situations." They mapped out a plan which called for a drastic narrowing of all their social activities, to be accomplished gradually to prevent attracting undue attention, withdrawal continuing until they could go to the United States for surgery. Meanwhile, only their most intimate friends and relatives were allowed to see the infant, and they were sworn to secrecy.

For a while, the Rodriguez's continued to attend some of the Sunday gatherings, but they no longer took their daughter. Now that they had a second child, whom they "could not take out in public," they felt that his absence would be too conspicuous if they took the little girl with them. Soon they avoided even these gatherings by taking the children every weekend to the country, where they remained in seclusion. During the two-week Carnival period and the Christmas holidays when there are many social functions and more than the usual amount of visiting, they left town to avoid "complicating situations."

There were special occasions, however, when they were obliged to receive visitors. The following incident made them realize the risk they ran "with curious and meddlesome people." One evening while entertaining guests, Dr. and Mrs. Rodriguez were momentarily absent from the living room when Francisco appeared. As they returned, they saw one of the visitors lifting the boy's hair to examine his deformity. This so upset them that thereafter he was never allowed out of their sight. They decided to see none but their closest friends and relatives and curtailed going to church as well.

The Rodriguez's endeavored to anticipate the inevitable time when Francisco would ask questions about his ear. As soon as he was old enough, his father told him that in a few years they would take him to New York City where he would have a "new ear made." When he reached school age, a home tutor was engaged. His father felt that if he allowed the boy to go to school, others might tease him and he would "come home complaining," or "maybe he would not like school." He was told, "When your bad little ear is fixed, you will be able to go to school with the other children, too." Sometimes he would stand in front of the mirror and examine his tiny lobe. He would ask his mother when he was going to have his "bad little ear" fixed. And she would say to him, "Very soon, but never mention it to your father for it upsets him too much to hear about it and he does not want you to speak of it."

While Francisco never mentioned his deformity to his father, and seldom to his mother, he was well aware of his parents' desire to conceal it from others. On trains he always sat in the corner and tried to remain as inconspicuous as possible. When the wind blew, he would press his head close to the seat, so no one would notice his defect. "We were always afraid someone might notice," his father explained, "and their startled expression at seeing something ugly or disagreeable would have made us suffer very much. And it might also hurt the boy."

When the time came for Francisco to wear short hair and suits customary for boys his age, his parents continued to dress him in the blouses and knee trousers of a 4- or 5-year-old. They taught him to reply if questioned: "I like it this way." If Dr. Rodriguez were asked why he kept his son's hair long, he would answer: "I wore my hair that way when I was his age and my wife wants the boy to do likewise. It's just an idiosyncrasy of hers." The mother and sister would give similar replies.

To prevent Francisco from becoming "effeminate," Dr. Rodriguez spent all of his free time teaching him exercises and games "to make him strong and manly." He taught him to ride horseback and shamed him if he fell off and cried. "The boy and I have become very close companions," his father explained. "He is so devoted to me he telephones me at my office just to talk to me, and sometimes I have to tell his mother to make him stop as it interferes with my work. If I come home late at night I have to go to his room and speak to him, or he won't go to sleep. He wants to grow up to be just like me."

During those years, Francisco's parents were so unhappy about his deformity, so distressed by the thought of the normal life he was missing, and the suffering he must endure in order to have an ear made, that they did everything they could to make up to him for it. Consequently, he was constantly waited upon, particularly by his father, who even helped him on with his overcoat. Francisco's wishes were granted whenever possible, for "we hated to deny him anything when he had such a great disadvantage." Occasionally he was punished when he behaved "too badly," but not as often as if he didn't "have this difficulty."

Clara, on the other hand, was disciplined and her parents were strict with her "because she has no handicap, and more is expected of her." But she resented the limitations imposed upon her. She was not permitted to bring friends home from school because they would see Francisco, and she could play only with her cousins. For a long time she had wanted a bicycle and skates like her other friends, but her father refused her anything that would take her out on the streets with other children while Francisco remained indoors. She became rebellious and said she didn't see why she had to suffer because of Francisco. Only once, to pacify Clara, Dr. Rodriguez let his wife take both children to a picnic. But Mrs. Rodriguez returned in such a nervous state due to her fear that someone would notice the boy's deformity or comment upon his clothes or hair that the experiment was not repeated.

It had become increasingly apparent to Clara that her brother usually got his own way and was the main object of their attention. Resenting this favoritism, she sometimes grew so angry that she fought with him and called him "hembrita" (little female), or "coronita" (little crown), although she was severely punished for it. By the age of 10 she had become sulky, argumentative, and jealous. Her father attributes the temperamental differences in his children to "their natural dispositions."

Francisco had three operations, but many months were to pass before the work on his ear could be completed. Between surgical procedures he wore a dressing on the side of his head. His hair had been cut, to his great pleasure, and he was allowed to wear long trousers. Since people no longer stared, the family could go out freely. If anyone remarked on Francisco's bandage, they said simply that he had had an operation.

All the family, except Francisco, were highly apprehensive about the operations and his brief periods of hospitalization. Dr. Rodriguez worried so that he lost weight. More than before, the parents felt that they had to "try to compensate" for their son's sufferings. They told him that when he had his "new ear," they could all return to Venezuela and take part in things they had missed before; that he would be able to go to school and picnics just as other children do. Both children were promised bicycles and skates as soon as they got home. But Francisco looked forward to something quite special: As he said to his mother, "Now that my ear will be fixed it will be nice to go home and have a boyfriend of my own."

Long before Francisco was aware that he was different from others, his parents' fear of society's attitude caused them to alter their lives and social relationships in order to prevent discovery of his defective ear. The seclusion they sought in expeditions to the country, their fabricated excuses, and their manner of dressing him were techniques to "protect" Francisco from gossip and ridicule. At the same time, however, they were shielding themselves, especially Dr. Rodriguez, who viewed his son's imperfection as a reflection upon his own machismo. Pride, fear of losing status and prestige, and feelings of shame all operated in their decision to keep the boy's deformity a secret.[9]

Other facts, too, stand out in sharp relief. Bound together by their "secret" and their mutual fear of discovery, the Rodriguez family presented a united front wherever they went. Yet among themselves the same phenomenon influenced and directed certain patterns of behavior that affected their relationships with each other.

Both parents, highly distressed about their son, centered attention on him, almost to the exclusion of their daughter. Markedly anxious about the son's deformity, Dr. Rodriguez developed a stronger emotional attachment to Francisco than his attachment to his wife and daughter. Furthermore, the boy's overdependence and reciprocal affection enhanced the father's ego satisfaction.

The sister, hurt and resentful of the restraints imposed upon her by her brother's plight and the favoritism shown him, grew jealous, moody, and antagonistic, alternately withdrawing into herself or turning toward her mother. Her own self-attitudes and those she will have in the future are, and will be, in large part the result of her particular relationships with the members of the family.

---

[9] We do not know what hidden factors may have been involved in determining their behavior. But many parents feel that somehow they are to blame for a deformed child. A sense of guilt sometimes drives them to resort to self-deprivation and other measures that may not be in the best interests of either the victim or his family, though they may think so. It is a form of penance of which they may be totally unaware.

Having spent his entire eight years with a family whose concerted efforts were to shelter him, Francisco had never felt the full impact of social prejudice. He was, consequently, the best adjusted in the family. Although aware that his defective ear was something the family wished to conceal, he expressed less concern about it than about his hair and clothes which, as he grew older, he realized were different from those of other children. Restrained from participation in primary configurations other than his family, he had no opportunity to establish relations with other individuals or to develop roles and attitudes with reference to them—important elements in the socialization process and the development of responsibility and self-confidence. Nor was there any provision by which he could free himself of the strong, emotionally toned and close identification with his father to direct his attention to a wider range of individuals.

What ultimate effects these years will have on the child's personality remain to be seen. It seems safe to assume, however, that Francisco will be forced to make many adjustments when he is finally allowed to participate with others. Not only has he had no opportunity to engage in the maturing social processes of cooperation or competition outside the family, but he has been the object of extraordinary protection, attention, and indulgence. Sooner or later, he is bound to meet critical situations for which he is totally unready, in which it will be impossible for his family to interpose themselves between him and the situation at hand. Furthermore, he has not been prepared for the abnormal-looking ear he is going to have. How sensitive he will be because of past conditioning experiences and the kind of interaction he had with the members of his family is conjectural. His parents, while accepting on an intellectual level the fact that his ear will never look normal, are emotionally unprepared for anything less than perfection. Francisco therefore thinks and plans in terms of a "new ear," not in terms of an imperfect one. All these considerations, then, combined with the child's overdependence on his father, are likely to produce a crisis when he is finally freed from the social isolation in which he has always been made to live.

In conclusion, it must be remembered that the manner in which the Rodriguez family responded to Francisco's deformity was not due simply to attitudes peculiar only to themselves but reflected the prevailing sociocultural attitudes toward facial deformities. In addition, the influence of specific Venezuelan cultural patterns must be taken into account in judging the kinds of adjustment and accommodation the family members made to their situation.

CHAPTER SIX

Surgery: The Patient
and the Surgeon

THE STRESS OF RECONSTRUCTIVE SURGERY*

> My face is like a nightmare that haunts me
> every minute of night and day; and even when
> I don't see it, I still feel its grotesque ugliness.
> (a patient)

So closely is the face tied to the core of the self and the sense
of identity that any visible damage to it, minimal or severe, is
normally accompanied by a pervading sense of shame and loss.
The victim wants to hide his defect and to avoid being looked at
—a reaction that reflects the symbolic values society attaches to
the face and that are implicit in such terms as "shamefaced," "face
the world," "lose face," and "face value." Grievously damaging
to his ego are the pity, curiosity, or revulsion that others manifest
at the sight of him and that are not only demoralizing but in many
cases seriously disorganizing in their effect on him and his life
situation.

The initial reaction to any damage to the face is commonly
one of acute distress, which may be followed by periods of
mourning and prolonged depression. Aware as he is of the de-
valuative attitude of society toward those whose faces are marred
or unsightly, the patient tends to carry over and ascribe the same
attitude to himself. Depending on his personal reactions to those
with facial deviations, prior to his own disfigurement, he antici-
pates scrutiny, rejection, or pity.

To the extent that the victim of facial trauma detects shock or
sorrow in the eyes of those around him, his self-devaluation and
sense of loss will deepen. Even before he sees himself in a mirror
he may receive clues as to the degree of damage. "From the way
my face felt, and the daily attention I received from specialists

* See Notes at back of book.

brought in for consultation," said Ingrid de Valery (Chapter One), "I knew my face was ruined. And there were the things I overheard—the nurses saying 'poor girl'—and the tone of extreme pity in the voices of my family and friends. There was no doubt in my mind as to what had happened. I felt dead inside." And a young war victim whose jaw had been shot away said: "I can still remember the look my lieutenant gave me when I was carried past him. That look froze me and filled me with panic."

So psychologically traumatizing is the sight of a disfigured face that it is not unusual for the victim of severe injury to entertain thoughts of suicide or drastic alterations of life plans. As Ingrid described her situation, "When I first saw myself in the mirror, I decided I could do one of three things. I could kill myself; I could enter a cloister, where I would be hidden from the world and could work; or I could go back into the world I knew and begin another life as an ugly woman."

In individuals who have a history of emotional instability, disfigurement may precipitate a crippling neurosis. A 24-year-old medical student who had a history of colitis and nervousness became an invalid following unsuccessful attempts to reconstruct her nose, which had been badly mutilated by an explosion while she was living abroad. When she came to the United States, she remained a recluse for two years, obsessed by her distorted appearance and the surgical scars on her arm and forehead, and fearful lest people think she was a "victim of lues." In addition, she complained of numbness in her legs, migraine headaches, upset stomach, fatigue, and nightmares—all of which she recognized as psychosomatic manifestations. To facilitate breathing and prevent further contracture of scar tissue, tubes were inserted into her nostrils. But to her this was a minor problem. "I wouldn't care if I couldn't breathe well my whole life. It's the way I look that matters. It's on my mind all the time. I suffer tremendous fatigue and have such anxiety facing people. I'm afraid of new people and I won't go anywhere." Several months of psychotherapy were necessary before her request for corrective surgery could be considered.

But there are also individuals who despite conspicuous disfigurement show extraordinary fortitude from the beginning in their determination to go on as before. Irrespective of attendant psychological mechanisms, such as denial, fantasy, and feelings of omnipotence, the assault upon the ego is so unrelenting that, once they have left the protective walls of the hospital, resistance is difficult to maintain. For example, the war victim mentioned above was satisfied with what the surgeons had accomplished, considering the extent of the original injury. Although further surgery would be required to improve both the appearance and the functional impairment of his mouth, he left the hospital in high anticipation of returning to his family and resuming his normal life. "I was not self-conscious at all," he said, "except when eating—and I knew that I would be fixed up soon." But the actual reality testing in the outside world quickly dampened his optimism. First there were his sister's tears when she saw him—and the pronounced dismay of his parents—to which he responded by trying to make light of his deformity. Then there were the reactions of people on the streets "I had not counted on the curiosity of men when I thought of coming back to normal life." Although he tried to ignore their pity, remarks, and glances, a series of unpleasant incidents finally forced him to stay home until such time as he would be "completely repaired."

While withdrawal and self-imposed isolation are more typical responses of persons with conspicuous facial damage, in rare instances the reaction and adjustment may be the converse of those just described.

James M. had had a history of personality disorganization and social maladjustment for most of his 22 years. Psychological disturbance in the army, gambling, drinking, desertion, and non-support of his wife, and suspected homosexuality had characterized the years preceding his accident. Then an angry acquaintance threw acid in his face, causing irreversible scarring, the loss of one eye, and part of an ear. Surprisingly James showed no evidence of depression—a reaction that had been anticipated. Following temporary discharge from the hospital and between readmissions, he set about reorganizing his life to the extent of returning to his wife and becoming more responsible and conforming. He explained his changed behavior thus: His whole family had been "jinxed" in one way or another before and since leaving Ireland.

Bad luck pursued them, but this accident, he said, had "ended the family jinx and from now on things will be better." Rationalizing or not, he was able to give adversity a unique and hopeful twist.

Theoretically, rehabilitation of the disfigured person begins when he enters the hospital. Plans include surgery and, if indicated, prosthetic aids, teaching, and vocational training. The goal is to return the patient to his family, job, and society. But the path to rehabilitation is often long and complicated. Healing processes for any given surgical procedure differ among individuals, and in correcting a primary defect the surgeon may be obliged to create a secondary one. Predictions of esthetic results are difficult to make, for there are limitations to what even the most skillful surgeon can achieve.

Many variables that contribute to success or failure in rehabilitating the facially disfigured are not necessarily related to the extent of surgical repair or restoration but rather to the patient's emotional and psychological makeup and his perception of his situation. Surgeons' definitions and interpretations of "success" and "failure" therefore may differ from those of the patient. Although function may be restored, enabling him to eat, or to speak, or to close his eyes, if the cosmetic results do not restore his self-image and provide him with the anonymity he craves, "success" from his standpoint is not achieved. To the degree that he evokes deprecating reactions he remains stigmatized.

Long-term or multistaged procedures can be especially demoralizing. Both hospitalization and surgical procedures, whether simple or complicated, normally produce anxiety. In addition to apprehension about physical pain and days of immobilization and discomfort, there are the uncertainty and concern about the esthetic outcome, for on the outcome the patient feels his future way of life may depend. Improvement may not be immediately noticeable. Indeed, he may look even worse during serial surgery.[1]

There may be several noticeable transformations or alterations in appearance thus creating for many persons a problem in self-

[1] For example, in situations requiring extensive skin grafting, tubed pedicle flaps, or exenteration of an orbit.

identity—"Who am I?"—and a serious disturbance of body image. As one patient put it, "No other form of physical injury presents these ever-changing imageries. There is a kaleidoscopic transformation in actual appearance. Is my image the image of the way I was born, is it the original disfigurement, or the one following the first operation, the tenth or the twentieth operation?"[2]

After each phase of the overall plan of reconstructive surgery, time is required for healing before an evaluation of progress can be made and further steps planned. During intermediate waiting periods that can extend into weeks or months, patients may alternate between hope and black despair. Imprisoned behind the shocking facade of a forehead flap, a temporary appliance, or suffering the indignity and humiliation of drooling or speech impairment, patients find the normal pursuits of society intolerable and remain in seclusion. Rage, frustration, and discouragement beset them, feelings frequently reinforced by their families, who, like the patients, have had no conception of the problems, complications, and time involved in facial restoration. When just so much can be accomplished at each successive stage, with no dramatic improvement, patients become despondent. Remarks such as these are common:

You keep thinking "just one more operation," and then afterwards you get discouraged because you don't look so different.
I don't think I can take any more.
The whole process of facial reconstruction is slow and tedious. It exhausts the patient physically and emotionally, and it requires courage and willpower to endure.
It is truly a common struggle of the surgeon, the patient, and the nurses.

For the person who must accept a prosthetic device designed to conceal or replace a lost part of the face, adjustment is difficult and emotionally taxing. Besides the deep psychological implications

[2] Although some studies have been made of the impact on the body image following physical injury, and of individuals' ability or inability to incorporate or integrate the change in the appearance of the body, an important and as yet unexplored area for research concerns those who experience multiple alterations in facial appearance. Not only are they confronted by a series of traumata emanating from within but, from the impact of their changed appearance, upon others as well.

of a prosthesis for the integrity of the body and the self-image, there is the fear of being unmasked should the appliance become dislodged, and the dread of being seen by another during its removal. "Most devastating to me," said a patient with a nasal prosthesis, "is the removal and replacement of my appliance. I am terrified someone will see the way I really look."

Throughout the often long and complicated struggle toward total rehabilitation, a high degree of motivation is essential. To help the patient maintain it, the support and understanding of the surgeon, staff, relatives, and friends are of inestimable value. Essential also to achieving optimal results in a long-term rehabilitation program is the cooperative effort of patient and surgical team.

COMMUNICATION AND INTERPERSONAL RELATIONS

The very nature of surgery as a speciality requires of potential and practicing surgeon alike that they give priority to the technical and medical–surgical aspects of each case. What is the immediate problem to be tackled? What surgical procedure is indicated to repair, reconstruct, or alter that part of the body which is distressing to the patient?

The training of interns and residents in surgery, in contrast to that in other medical specialities, is perforce concerned with gaining experience and developing skills in the operating room. Because close personal relationships with surgical patients tend to be viewed as only slightly, if at all, relevant to success in diagnosis and treatment as compared, for example, to their importance in the practice of internal medicine, the social, psychological, and cultural determinants of the patient's perception of his situation—his fears, needs, expectations, and emotional state—receive little attention in the training program.

It has been observed that surgery as a career speciality is chosen by persons predisposed toward action and challenged by the intricate technological aspects of procedures to solve or ameliorate problems, in preference to specialties requiring close social interchange and communication with patients. Whether it is the result of the educational program or the orientation and values of the surgeon trainee—and there is evidence that these all play a part—the fact remains that in general the young surgeon perceives the doctor–patient relationship as peripheral to the role and function of a surgeon.[3]

In reality, however, success in management, treatment, and rehabilitation of the disfigured patient is determined in no small measure by the kind of relationship established between him and his doctor. Mutual trust and respect and clear lines of communication are essential ingredients both for preparing the patient psychologically for surgery and for maintaining a sound relationship with him until he is discharged. This ideal objective is not always achieved. Some patients are hard to handle. There are those who vacillate—who are late for or do not keep their appointments. Others fail to comply with the prescribed medical regimen. Some are demanding and complain constantly, or become recalcitrant or even hostile. Others may discharge themselves from the hospital or fail to go through with planned additional procedures. Strain, misunderstanding, even open conflict may arise between patients and staff members, or between patient and surgeon; communication may break down altogether.

When such situations occur, the surgeon understandably is frustrated. He may become irritated, discouraged, even disgusted. In all likelihood he will label the patient "uncooperative," "stubborn," or a "personality problem." Regarding his behavior as difficult, deviant, or seemingly inappropriate, the surgeon tends to interpret it from a psychological perspective, as an idiosyncratic feature of his personality. He may refer him to a social worker or a psychiatrist, whose psychological orientation (frequently Freudian) leads them to focus on the personality and to interpret behavior in terms of repression, hostility, guilt, neurosis, psychosis, and the like. While it is true that deviant behavior may be symptomatic of an underlying emo-

[3] Kutner, Bernard, "Surgeons and Their Patients: A Study in Social Perception," in *Patients, Physicians and Illness*, edited by E. Gartly Jaco. The Free Press, Glencoe, Illinois, 1958, pp. 384–397.

tional disturbance, it is equally true—and more often than is generally recognized—that the explanations are to be found on cultural and social levels.

Particularly in large urban centers where the character of the patient population is heterogeneous, surgical services are likely to be dispensed across boundaries of ethnicity and social class. As a consequence, patients represent a wide range of sociocultural differences that play an important role in their reactions to illness and hospitalization and their attitudes and responses toward management, treatment, and rehabilitation. If these differences are neither understood nor taken into account, the management and therapeutic outcome may be adversely affected.[4] This is demonstrated in the following case:

Arturo G. was born and reared in Spain but for the past nine years had been a university instructor in the United States. Several months before consulting a plastic surgeon he had incurred multiple facial scars as a result of a motorboat accident. They extended over the right side of his nose, leaving an indentation in his right cheek and the right frontal temporal region, with some scarring of his eyelids.

The first operation involved excising and suturing the scar over the right temporal region. The surgeon's next concern was repairing the markedly damaged nose. But Mr. G. declined the operation on the grounds that the correction of his nose could be postponed. "What bothers me the most," he said, "is the sagging of my eyelid. It seems as though my eyes have lost their sparkle and life. The importance of the eyes lies in their brilliance and what they convey to another, and mine look tired and 'blah.' "

In view of the esthetic contrast between the slight eye defect and the conspicuous nasal scars, the patient's attitude was, from the surgeon's frame of reference, unrealistic and bizarre. On the basis of a personality evaluation by a psychiatrist, Mr. G. was

[4] Macgregor, Frances Cooke, *Social Science in Nursing: Applications for the Improvement of Patient Care.* Russell Sage Foundation, New York, 1960.

diagnosed as having an obsessive character disorder, with narcissistic tendencies. Considered in the context of his social and cultural milieu, however, his reaction was not strange. In Spain, the eyes have special social significance. Described by Cervantes as "silent tongues," to the Spaniard they play a predominant role in communication, particularly in flirtations, when much signaling is done with them. They are "the windows of the soul"—so much so that the Spaniard is said to be far more affected by the quality of the gaze than he is by the color of the eyes.[5] The high value of the eyes as distinct from other facial features was the decisive element in Mr. G.'s reaction and accounted for the difference in priority accorded the surgical procedures by him and his surgeon. . . .

As important as the patients' cultural background is the role played by social class in behavior and interpersonal relations. By and large, members of the health professions derive from the middle class, and their expectations of how patients "should" behave reflect their own standards and values. Hence they sometimes become irritated or impatient when dealing with lower-class patients whose attitudes do not conform to what is deemed proper or acceptable. In teaching hospitals, especially, where clinic patients tend to come from ethnic minorities and lower socioeconomic levels, the status gap between surgeon and patient is apt to be wide. Consequently, misunderstandings and problems of communication are frequent. Physicians—particularly surgeons—are regarded with awe, and in their presence, besides feeling apprehensive, many lower-class patients, embarrassed by the marked disparities in formal education and socioeconomic status, become confused and inarticulate in their insecurity. Their failure to comply with expected middle-class modes of conduct and ritualized forms of courtesy sometimes leads medical personnel to compound misinterpretations and unfavorable judgments of them with the commonly held stereotypes of lower-

[5] Ellis, H., *The Soul of Spain*. Houghton Mifflin, Boston, 1931.

class patients as unintelligent and shiftless because they are poor or do not speak "good" English.

Emotional rather than intellectual reactions to patients not only affect the therapeutic relationship adversely but may influence the decision to accept or reject candidates for surgery, as the following incident illustrates:

At a clinic evaluation attended by some fifteen surgeons, residents, and nurses, a discussion was held about a 16-year-old black girl who sat rolling her eyes and chewing gum while various members examined her deformity. At the end of the conference, during which no one had spoken directly to her, she left the room without looking at anyone or saying good-bye. Her demeanor had struck one young surgeon as arrogant and hostile. Said he heatedly: "If we were to operate on her, she'd always be a problem. The insolence of the lower classes makes it impossible for me to deal with them. My private Negro patients are middle-class. *They* say 'thank you.' They keep their appointments. But lower-class people are belligerent. They don't thank you. They don't come back for follow-ups or keep their appointments. *I* certainly wouldn't operate on her."

In their studies of doctor–patient relationships, social scientists have observed that the doctor's perception of the patients' socioeconomic status—and the level of knowledge and other characteristics he associates with it—influences to a considerable degree the amount of time he spends with them and what and how much he tells them about treatment, possible complications, and prognosis. Because education is often equated with intelligence and the capacity to adjust, patients perceived as being middle- or upper-class are more likely to be credited with ability to understand medical explanations, whereas the comprehension of the less educated, particularly if lower-class, is more likely to be underrated.

For example, a study aimed at measuring physicians' judgments about patients in an outpatient clinic showed that, of 89 doctors, 81 percent tended to underestimate the level of knowledge of the clinic patient population. Those who seriously misjudged patients' knowledge tended to spend less time discussing the patients' problems with them than did those whose evaluations were more accurate.[6]

The effect upon the patient who receives only cursory information because he is perceived as ill-informed or unable to understand is to react "either by asking uninspired questions or refraining from questioning the doctor at all, thus reinforcing the doctor's view that the patient is ill-equipped to comprehend his problem, and further reinforcing the doctor's tendency to skirt discussion of the problem. Lacking guidance by the doctor, the patient performs at a low level; hence, the doctor rates his capacities as even lower than they are."[7]

Although the findings of the above study were not conclusive, they substantiate my observations of the interaction between plastic surgeons and patients: namely, that the patient who is given a thorough explanation throughout the stages of his treatment tends not only to participate more actively and effectively with the surgeon but is more likely to accept the plans and goals for rehabilitation.

THE PATIENT AS A PERSON

Sources of patients' apprehension, dissatisfaction, and/or hostility, or their lack of cooperation in treatment and rehabilitation can often be controlled if medical and nursing personnel are sensitized to the psychological effects of treatment and management. More often than one might suspect, those aspects of their surgical experiences that patients find most disturbing and tend to remember longest are not the surgical procedures per se but the particular commissions or omissions in their management.

During hospital rounds and clinic evaluation of patients, physicians routinely discuss in the patients' presence the disfigurements and possible surgical procedures. Important as this practice is for teaching purposes, it is for many patients a

[6] Pratt, L., A. Seligman, and G. Reader, "Physicians' Views on the Level of Medical Information Among Patients," in *Patients, Physicians and Illness*, edited by E. Gartly Jaco, op. cit., pp. 225–226.

[7] Ibid., p. 226.

frightening, if not a psychologically traumatic experience. To most people, especially those of certain cultural and ethnic backgrounds, a hospital is a place to be avoided if possible. Even when a patient comes to the hospital clinic to request an operation, he regards the idea of surgery with all it implies—the anesthetic, "being cut," pain, and so on—with varying degrees of dread.

While the patient under consideration may be sitting quietly in the examining chair, expressionless and seemingly unperturbed, it is often forgotten that he is highly sensitive to every word or sign that has, or that he thinks has, reference to him. Technical language, although certainly preferable to an alarming lay vocabulary, can (by the very fact that it is technical and, to most, incomprehensible) cause some patients to conclude that their cases involve potential dangers which the doctors do not want them to know about. Discussion of surgical procedure, if interspersed with such anxiety-producing words as "incision," "scalpel," "detach," and "split" (not to mention the effect of tones of voice, facial expressions, and gestures), may leave a painful and lasting impression. The effect of discussion in front of patients is illustrated by the reaction of an 18-year-old girl to hearing the plan of action for an operation to be performed on her nose that afternoon:

DOCTOR: "We'll expose everything here" (running his finger down patient's nose). Patient frowns.
DOCTOR: "We'll have to loosen everything." Patient recoils. (Doctor draws diagram of procedure on blackboard.) Patient puts hand over eyes to avoid seeing.
DOCTOR: "We'll use a Number 10 blade." Patient shudders. "We'll detach the flap and move the septal flap forward. We don't want to get a perforation."
SECOND DOCTOR (pointing to diagram): "I'd split it here and chisel the bone."

Following this conference the patient came to the sociologist's office, pale, with perspiration standing on her forehead. She had looked forward to the correction of her deformity but was now so shaken that she wished she "had never come here in the first place."

Signs of indecision and discussions in front of patients about alternative methods of treatment, or conflicting opinions among staff members not only heighten anxiety but may undermine the patient's confidence in the surgeon and his associates. In general, patients are not accustomed to and often misinterpret the technical dialogue, questions, and exchanges among surgeons and trainees about diagnoses and procedures that are routine features of teaching hospitals. The patient, hearing only part of what is said, and not understanding all, may become panic-stricken at the slightest comment or gesture, construing it as having dire implications.

CANDOR AND CONFIDENCE

Under any circumstances, the sight of one's own face, surgically mutilated, is a shock that can be compounded by the outcome and the residual effects, especially if the patient has not been forewarned. For example, when radical surgery is indicated, the patient should be as thoroughly prepared as possible for whatever extent of disfigurement and improvement can be anticipated:

A patient was told no more than that because of a malignant growth he would have to have his eye removed. Although he was devastated by the thought of losing his eye, his fear of cancer was even greater, and he readily agreed to an operation. He said he assumed that his eye would be replaced by an artificial one. He underwent an exenteration of the orbit and resection of the jaw, necessary to eradicate the cancer. On his third postoperative day he went to the bathroom. "When I saw myself in the mirror, I screamed," he said. "I realized I was looking into my own skull. I thought, 'Heavenly Father! What have I done?' . . . Then when I asked the surgeon about a prosthetic eye, he said, 'You can't have one—you have no socket.' Just like that! I said, 'My God, how am I going to live? How am I going to work again?'" An additional and unexpected blow was the discovery that he would be deprived of his upper denture for some time because of the delay in the preparation of the palatal defect and the construction of necessary prosthetic devices. This complication prevented his returning to his job, even though the orbital cavity was concealed by a patch. Totally unprepared for these surgical sequelae, he went into a severe depression. When seen a year later, he was bitter about the management of his case, viewing the withholding of information as a betrayal. "I hate that hospital," he said. "I'll never go back there again!"

The deliberate minimizing of a patient's disfigurement in an effort to spare him further pain often only serves to increase the traumatizing effect when he sees himself in the mirror for the first time.

A 45-year-old truck driver was severely burned on the face, hands, and body in a highway crash, in which he also lost his hair, eyelashes, and part of his right ear. He was taken to a small hospital. Although he knew he was hurt, he did not realize how badly. "I kept thinking to myself," he said, " 'it won't be too long and I'll be out of here.' " The demeanor of the hospital personnel contributed to his optimism. "Everybody stopped in to see me—nurses from other floors, when they went off duty— doctors on their way to see other patients. They all seemed to say: 'Don't worry—everything will be fixed in no time at all.' The doctors said: 'Don't worry, we'll get you fixed up again.' "

The patient had planned to be married soon, and even while in the hospital he continued with the arrangements. One day when a nurse had him in a wheelchair, he insisted that he could go to the bathroom alone—the first time he had been on his feet long enough to do so. Worried because he didn't come out, the nurse went in after him. She found him frozen in front of the mirror. He was seeing himself for the first time since the accident—"I'm a Frankenstein. That's what I am! I'm a monster!" he cried. He called off his marriage and never spoke of it again. Later, recalling the shock of seeing himself, he said: "I had no idea I was that bad off. The bottom dropped out of my stomach. I felt like— you know—bang!"—putting his hand to his temple, he pulled an imaginary trigger. "I knew everything I was used to at the time was gone. My good times are over. I know that."[8]

[8] Schoepf, Brooke, personal communication.

Another roadblock often encountered by medical personnel stems from the patients' exaggerated expectation of what plastic surgery can do for them. The miracles that are attributed to plastic surgery, not to mention the "amazing transformations in personality" that are also reported, have unfortunately given the general public an impression of achievements that are not always commensurate with the facts. Even medically sophisticated laymen sometimes have unrealistic beliefs and expectations about the wonders plastic surgery can accomplish. In relatively reputable magazines such titles as "How to Get a New Face," and "New Faces, New Lives," convey the notions that scars can be completely eradicated, broken faces repaired "like new," and birthmarks erased with ease. Not realized are the potential complications and problems in surgical restoration and reconstruction and in the making and fitting of prostheses. In addition, there is the possibility of developing keloids[9] (especially in persons with dark skin) and the difference in color and texture that can result from skin grafting. These and other conditions can prevent achievement of the perfection desired by the patients, even when surgery is performed by the most skilled doctors.

The patient's concept of a successful cosmetic outcome may be quite different from what the surgeon assumes and indeed may even exceed what the surgeon knows is possible. What can and cannot be accomplished should be made crystal clear to the patient and if risks must be run or technical problems make the outcome uncertain, he should be told in advance to give him the advantage of being forewarned and of participating in all the final decisions.

There will be instances, however, when full presentation of facts and acknowledgment by surgeons of doubtful results will not be *heard* by the patient, so convinced is he of success. In his wishful thinking, he endows the surgeon with omnipotent powers. One determined patient, for example, resisted all efforts by the residents and the chief surgeon to impress upon her the questionable outcome of a second operation, which she was certain would eradicate her residual scars. Fixing her attention on

---

[9] A thick scar resulting from excessive growth of fibrous tissue.

the rows of surgical books in the room where she was being interviewed, she said, "But I'm just sure the doctors will succeed. Look at all those books, and think how much they know!"

TALKING AND LISTENING TO PATIENTS

More often than is generally recognized, patients' dissatisfaction and the litigations that sometimes develop are traceable to the surgeon's lack of concern for and interest in the patient as a person. Whether the disfigurement is mild or severe, in seeking surgical help the patient is also asking for acceptance and understanding of his problem and fears. "He listens to you," "He takes time to explain things," are commendations of physicians that carry positive weight with today's increasingly medically sophisticated public, which looks for compassion as well as competence.

A brusque or hurried manner on the surgeon's part generates frustration and despair—even resentment, should the operative and postoperative course be less than smooth. On the other hand, as Meyer points out: "An enduring grudge reaction that settles on the physician or surgeon can almost never breed in an atmosphere where genuine, unhurried attempts to appreciate the patient as an individual person have been made, when the operative and postoperative situations have been fully explained, and when the patient, though disappointed, knows he has been treated with respect and concern."[10]

Of particular importance during the long and often arduous course of multiple surgical procedures is consistently to allow the patient to express himself freely. By doing so the surgeon gives him a sense of support and acceptance through which he can gain some strength to withstand his affliction. Refusal to discuss his feelings of discouragement or hopelessness, on the other hand, may actually intensify these sentiments rather than mitigate them.

[10] Meyer, Eugene, "Psychiatric Aspects of Plastic Surgery," in *Reconstructive Plastic Surgery*, vol. 1, *General Principles*, edited by John M. Converse. W. B. Saunders Company, Philadelphia, 1964, p. 371.

Also of therapeutic importance is the support provided by ancillary personnel. Although all treatment facilities for plastic surgery patients do not include psychological investigation or counseling, their problems are no less complicated than those of other handicapped persons, and such services should be considered. Many teaching hospitals today have professionals trained in psychiatry, psychology, and social work who conduct group therapy sessions in which patients with similar disabilities can talk out their mutual problems. Such measures, it has been found, can often help to sustain patients' morale, give support, and provide outlets for hostility and frustration.[11]

Despite the remarkable achievements of modern plastic surgery, a face that has sustained severe damage to soft tissue and bone structure can seldom be restored to its original appearance. Even with surgical or prosthetic modifications the results may be far from ideal in the eyes of either doctor or patient. When nothing further can be gained by continuing surgical procedures, the physical phase of rehabilitation may be considered completed. The possibility that in the unforeseeable future new techniques or discoveries may offer new hope is beside the point. The fact remains that, as far as can be determined in the light of current knowledge, the patient is left with a lasting residual disfigurement.

Psychological rehabilitation then becomes the major goal. If from the beginning the patient has been prepared for the limitations of the surgical procedures that possibly will fall short of his expectations, it will help to cushion the shock of the inevitability of permanent damage. Nevertheless, so long as a patient is required to return for further evaluation and surgical consideration, his hopes will continue to be bolstered.

An essential phase in the rehabilitation of any handicapped person is that of coming to terms with and accepting his disability. Withholding or avoidance of the facts in an effort to spare him further suffering is for the most part motivated by

[11] There is some evidence that patients who are facially disfigured are not receptive to group sessions. More research is essential before using this technique.

humanitarian concern, but in the long run it may not be in his best interest. While hope and optimism are important psychological crutches in the face of adversity, to conceal information that he will eventually discover for himself is to delay or interfere with the process of rehabilitation. In the case of parents of a disfigured child, however, it may be necessary to pace the giving of facts with their readiness to assimilate them.[12]

The surgeon's reluctance to present the patient with the facts is sometimes unconsciously motivated by his need to avoid a painful experience. He rationalizes his sidestepping on the grounds that it is best for the patient. "We must not eliminate the element of hope," said one surgeon in explanation of his evasive response to a patient's questions about future possibilities. "It is better to leave the patient with some doubt about further improvement. Let him discover (the futility of additional surgery) slowly."

"Leaving the door open" for whatever reasons is sufficient justification for many patients to postpone the immediate task of constructively coping with reality. One teen-ager, for example, delayed entering college for two successive years because he insisted upon waiting for the completion of experimentation from which, his surgeon had said, *might* evolve a technique that could eventuate in the boy's improvement.

There are no unequivocal rules about what and how much to tell patients. Decisions must be made on an individual basis. In special circumstances the removal of all hope could be psychologically disastrous. In general, however, as studies of psychological adjustment to physical handicaps have shown, the mature individual is both capable and desirous of knowing the facts. The sooner he comes to terms with and accepts his situation, the more likely he is to begin the work of adjustment.[13]

[12] Davis, Fred, *Passage Through Crisis: Polio Victims and Their Families.* Bobbs-Merrill, Indianapolis, 1963.
[13] Wright, Beatrice A., *Physical Disability: A Psychological Approach.* Harper and Bros., New York, 1960; also Davis, op. cit.

CHAPTER SEVEN

Some Dilemmas
of Cosmetic Surgery

THE DEMAND FOR COSMETIC SURGERY

> I am convinced that nothing has so marked an
> influence on the direction of a man's mind as
> his appearance, and not his appearance in itself
> so much as his conviction that it is attractive
> or unattractive.
>
> (Tolstoy, *Childhood*)

For some, the subject of cosmetic surgery may seem too frivolous
or trivial to warrant social scientific investigation. Compared
with the very real social and psychological problems of persons
who are severely disfigured, or for whom appearing in public is a
dreaded ordeal, such treatment needs as a face lifting, breast
augmentations, and rhinoplasties as matters for attention do
indeed seem unimportant.

Trivial as these may appear at first glance, however, the
growing requests for such procedures do have implications,
transcending the mere act of surgical alterations, that are of
great interest to the student of human behavior.

Cosmetic or "esthetic" surgery is described as surgery performed
in the attempt to improve the appearance of "normal" individuals, whereas "reconstructive" surgery refers to operations
undertaken to correct, as far as possible, the face or other parts
of the body that are distorted or maimed as a result of congenital
anomalies, disease, or trauma.

The legitimization of cosmetic surgery by American society in
general and the medical profession in particular is relatively
recent. Twenty-five years ago it was considered a novel procedure, an indulgence of the privileged, one usually sought covertly
and kept secret. To hide their identity women used pseudonyms
and subterfuge, and men who wanted their noses reshaped
attempted to conceal their real motives, even from the doctor,
behind complaints of functional disabilities such as difficulty in

breathing or nosebleeds.[1] For their part, surgeons tended to be suspicious of the "vain male," questioning his emotional stability and sometimes suggesting psychological clearance before agreeing to operate.

Today cosmetic surgery is enjoying what has been called a "cosmetic boom." Nearly 1 million Americans underwent operations in 1971, compared to some 15,000 in 1949.[2] The interest and the demand for external alterations and revisions are so great that, as a division of plastic surgery, cosmetic surgery has attained sufficient growth and specialization to boast its own national and international meetings. While there is still some bemusement and humorous stigma attached to having "nose jobs," breast augmentations, hair transplants, and similar "nonessential" procedures, disapproval has for the most part been dissipated as more and more people are convinced that their needs and aspirations are inextricably related to the way they look. So strong is this conviction that persons who would ordinarily cringe at the thought of going to the hospital are able to overcome their fears in anticipation of looking better.

Although cosmetic surgery is sometimes referred to as minor surgery, no surgery is in actuality minor. There is always some risk. Anesthesia, cutting, possible infection, and pain, not to mention the possibility of disappointing results, are to be considered. Yet applicants, young and old, from all walks of life— social, ethnic, and economic—are voluntarily *asking* to be operated on!

From a sociological perspective the current fascination with cosmetic surgery may be seen as a reflection of and a response to a variety of pressures, shifting values, and attitudinal changes. Aging, always unpleasant to contemplate, but nevertheless to be endured as gracefully as possible, has become a fearful prospect in a society that focuses inordinate attention on youth and

[1] Macgregor, Frances Cooke, and Bertram Schaffner, "Screening Patients for Nasal Plastic Operations: Some Sociologic and Psychiatric Considerations," *Psychosomatic Medicine*, vol. 12, no. 5, 1950, pp. 277–291.
[2] *New York Post*, September 7, 1971.

beauty, treats its old as social rejects, and denies death even to extending the "image of life" by cosmetic artifice.[3] Signs of aging, traditionally the bête noir of women, are now equally alarming to men. Obsolescence comes early these days in business and industry and the job lost at 40 may be the last job. Baggy eyes, jowls, bald heads, and double chins in a time of strong competition and job scarcity are real impediments.[4]

The sexual revolution, the preoccupation with eroticism, and the objectification of the body are also reflected both in the quantity and in the broadening spectrum of requests for cosmetic surgery. For example, more and more women are undergoing breast augmentation to attract and/or hold men whose ideal models are featured in such media as *Playboy*, *Esquire*, and underground films.[5] For the same purposes women ask for the removal of abdominal "stretch marks," sometimes telltale signs of childbearing.

In their wish to change their sexual identities male transsexuals and transvestites want tattooing eradicated and their noses, eyes, and cheeks altered to look more feminine. As for the middle-aged homosexual male, his motives for surgery are generally and frankly related to an excessive fear of looking old. Within the homosexual community emphasis on youth is said to be even greater than it is in society at large, and the crisis of aging comes earlier than it does in the heterosexual male. The latter's diminishing sexual attractiveness may be compensated for by a

---

[3] This is a matter of professional pride in the undertaking business. Hence the understandable pleasure of the undertaker who reported that after the many hours of work on the body of President Franklin D. Roosevelt, people remarked, ". . . he looks like his old self again and *much younger*" (italics added). Mitford, Jessica, *The American Way of Death*. Fawcett World Library, Crest Books, New York, 1964, p. 147.

[4] To qualify for an executive position in his firm a 35-year-old man was advised to have plastic surgery of his underdeveloped chin so that he might better fit the "corporate image."

[5] One young woman, married less than a year, requested breast augmentation to please her husband, whose ideal was Raquel Welch. "My poor husband said he never dated anybody under a 36B until he met me, and, gee, I'm a 32A and I think I ought to do something about it!"

wife and children, but the aging homosexual's life style is more severely affected by the visible ravages of age.[6]

Once a subject for gossip columnists and sly speculations, surgery for the enhancement of one's appearance is now fully legitimated. Amy Vanderbilt discusses on TV her delight with her face-lift, Phyllis Diller jokes about her new nose and smoothed-out wrinkles,[7] and Senator Proxmire unabashedly attends Congressional meetings with the not yet healed scars from his cosmetic surgery and a skull cap covering his new hair transplant.[8]

The recent rash of popular books and TV programs about the social and psychological rewards of such surface changes and rejuvenations has sparked a desire for plastic surgery in countless numbers of persons who might never have thought of it, as well as in those who have tried and failed to solve their problems by means ranging from psychiatry to encounter groups. Typical of the latter is the following letter:

Dear ———:

   I have just read of the help with surgery for cosmetic purposes in Dr. X's column. I am 48 years of age and recently forced out of my home, after 31 years of marriage and 31 years of hard back-breaking work, by a 30-year-old blonde worming her way into my husband's life. I left because of the degradation and heartache. I have joined clubs and Parents without Partners because I can't stand to be alone and feel life isn't worth much anymore. At my age, and not being endowed with natural beauty, I feel if I could even get some of the face lines removed it might restore some self-confidence and the will to live, which I seem to have lost along with the safe secure feeling of aging with dignity. Is there a good plastic surgeon on this coast you could recommend?

The popularity of certain types of surgical procedures not only reflects fads and fashions in facial esthetics, for example, in Europe the patrician-type nose of Princess Anne is said to be gaining favor over the "Jackie-Onassis-type nose" or the small

---

[6] Simon, William, and John H. Gagnon, "Homosexuality: The Formulation of a Sociological Perspective," *Journal of Health and Social Behavior*, vol. 8, no. 3, 1967, pp. 177–185.

[7] *New York Daily News*, February 8, 1972.

[8] *New York Post*, February 14, 1972.

turned-up nose,[9] but serves as a barometer of social and political trends. The "black is beautiful" movement and identification with Africa has instilled a growing pride in dark skin, Afro hair, and other Negroid characteristics to the extent that cosmetic surgeons are now advised to learn to provide African features for their black patients rather than the once favored Anglo-Saxon characteristics.[10] Similarly there is a rapidly growing militancy across the United States among young Jewish students who, manifesting a nationalistic pride and their identification with Israel and Zionism, are proclaiming that "Jewish is beautiful" and calling for Jews to maintain their Jewish identity.[11] Although difficult to document at this time, it is quite conceivable that the number of requests for rhinoplasties for the sole purpose of reducing one's visibility as a Jew will decline.

THE SURGEON'S DILEMMA*

The American medical profession's acceptance of cosmetic surgery as a therapeutic procedure is reflected in the growing number of plastic surgery clinics and health care plans that now make it possible for almost anyone to obtain partial or complete correction of a defect. With the advent of Medicaid, corrective procedures are available even to persons on welfare.

The changing attitudes toward cosmetic surgery and the increasing demands for it are results of several trends. Dominant among these are the high premium on physical attributes and the cultural pressure to conform coupled with a social climate in which one finds so many people plagued by a fear of loneliness, uncertainty, and a lack of self-identity. Additionally, there is the emphasis on youth—the current devaluation of those who are "over 30"—which, as noted above, exacts a heavy toll from the middle-aged and elderly with respect to employment.

* See Notes at back of book.
[9] *Time Magazine*, February 21, 1972.
[10] *Medical World News*, September 11, 1970.
[11] *The New York Times*, March 13, 1971.

Further impetus to the demand for cosmetic surgery has been given by the findings of scientific research on the social and psychological consequences of facial disfigurement: namely, that existing stereotypes—mostly denigrating or stigmatic—about the personality or character of one who has a receding chin, hook nose, malformed ears, or facial scars can adversely affect his mental health and life chances.

Although beneficial in many ways, the wide acceptance of cosmetic surgery has nonetheless accelerated its hazards and complications. The public today is sophisticated about medical care and the evaluation of its competence. When dissatisfied, patients are assertive of their rights and do not hesitate to seek legal aid. The plastic surgeon therefore is more vulnerable than ever. His difficulties are not necessarily related to surgical skill but lie in the area of human relations and communication. Dealing now as he must with a heterogeneous patient population, representing a wide range of sociocultural differences, the matter of correct evaluation and selection of candidates is beset with pitfalls both for him and his patients.

Unfortunately there exists no personality profile or statistical chart by which, computer-like, one can learn in seconds whether a patient will be a psychological risk: for instance, what his real motivation for surgery and unspoken expectations are, whether he will cooperate or pose a management problem, whether he will be punitive or litigious if things go wrong. At best, a personality profile is a concept that rests on normative assumptions, and while statistical frequency may be interpreted as statistically "normal," it does not follow that the patient is normal in a mental health sense. Even if one had a chart covering all types of personality with mathematical weighting of characteristics that, when submitted to statistical analysis, would indicate or contraindicate surgery, other variables (social class and ethnicity, for example) would still make such an instrument of dubious value.

Since lack of relevant information is one of the major causes not only of errors in evaluation but also of misunderstanding in the management of patients, it is important for the surgeon to try to know his patient. But to know him well enough to make a judicious decision with respect to surgery often takes more interviewing time than many surgeons feel is either possible or essential. It is assumed that when a cosmetic defect about which a patient complains is evident and operable, it is both unnecessary and unprofitable to investigate or discuss with him his problems, motives, and expectations. This assumption is erroneous. In contrast to the conspicuously disfigured patient, whose needs are situationally real and obvious, the one who presents a "minor" defect poses special problems.

THE PATIENT'S MOTIVES

As evidenced by research findings,[12] the patient with a slight defect tends to assess it as more conspicuous than it is and is also apt to be the most demanding. Also, the smaller the defect that troubles him, the more likely he is to focus on minute details and to magnify postoperatively any residual imperfections.

Cursory consultations with such patients seldom expose their underlying motives. Given reasons, such as wanting to look better and to get or hold a job or a spouse, are so highly sanctioned today as to obviate questioning. In many instances the stated reasons may be the real ones. But in as many others they can be oversimplifications or merely a lesser element in motivation.

It is not uncommon for the presenting complaints of patients with mild or moderate deformities to be symptomatic of emotional disturbance unrelated to the deformity.[13] In a psychiatric analysis of women seeking rhinoplasty, Meyer and his associates[14] concluded that preconscious and unconscious factors

---

[12] Macgregor, Frances Cooke, et al., *Facial Deformities and Plastic Surgery: A Psychosocial Study*. Charles C Thomas, Springfield, Illinois, 1953.

[13] Macgregor and Schaffner, "Screening Patients for Nasal Plastic Operations: Some Sociologic and Psychiatric Considerations," op. cit.

[14] Meyer, Eugene, et al., "Motivational Patterns in Patients Seeking Elective Plastic Surgery: I. Women Who Seek Rhinoplasty," *Psychosomatic Medicine*, vol. 22, no. 3, 1960, pp. 193–201.

play an important part in the motivation of patients, and interpretations of these center around the following: conflicts in
sexual identification; ambivalence in patients' identifications
with parents; the symbolic (sexual) meaning of the nose and the
wish for surgery; concepts of body image; and the incidence of
psychotherapy.

Some unstable individuals select one body part that they
claim to be deformed as an unconscious method of avoiding their
shortcomings of personality. They are convinced that this single
flaw causes all their problems and that plastic surgery will
magically transform their lives. In a study of 50 rhinoplasty
patients, Linn and Goldman[15] found a high incidence of neurosis,
whereas Jacobson et al.[16] found that the male patient seeking
surgery for mild congenital deformity is apt to suffer from serious emotional illness. As for mammoplasty, according to Knorr,
Hoopes, and Edgerton[17] many adolescent and adult females
who request breast augmentation exhibit hysterical character
traits and are prone to depression.

Besides the person who presents a single complaint, it is not
unusual for a patient obsessed with real or imagined defects to
shift attention from one body part to another and to move from
one surgeon to another seeking relief but, all too often, finding
disaster. In such cases, too, latent psychological disturbances that
have gone undetected may be triggered by the surgery, as in the
following case:*

A 43-year-old unmarried woman, dissatisfied with the results of
a surgically successful rhinoplasty, demanded a second operation
with the additional request that the wrinkles under her eyes be

* See Notes at back of book.

[15] Linn, Louis, and Irving B. Goldman, "Psychiatric Observations Concerning Rhinoplasty," *Psychosomatic Medicine*, vol. 11, no. 5, 1949, pp.
307–314.

[16] Jacobson, Wayne E., M. T. Edgerton, E. Meyer, A. Canter, and
R. Slaughter, "Psychiatric Evaluation of Male Patients Seeking Cosmetic
Surgery," *Plastic and Reconstructive Surgery*, vol. 26, no. 4, 1960, pp. 356–
372.

[17] Knorr, Norman J., J. E. Hoopes, and M. T. Edgerton, "Psychiatric-
Surgical Approach to Adolescent Disturbance in Self Image," *Plastic and
Reconstructive Surgery*, vol. 41, no. 3, 1968, pp. 248–253.

removed. Two lengthy interviews with her revealed that her complaints were symptomatic of serious mental and emotional illness. She was an attractive woman who endeavored to pass for 25 years of age. The defects of which she complained were so slight as hardly to be noticeable; yet, because of them she insisted that she had been unable to obtain work for a protracted length of time. She had had an unhappy childhood and adult life. In her view, her father was a reprehensible man and, like him, most men were exploiters. She was hostile and vindictive and blamed all her difficulties and poor interpersonal relationships on people and circumstances outside herself. She failed to see that her trouble in obtaining and holding jobs did not result from her appearance but from her own personality shortcomings and her obsession that she was being exploited and persecuted. In view of her disturbed condition it was recommended that her request for surgery be denied. At this the patient became extremely agitated and belligerent and insisted that the surgeon operate on her. When he refused, she then consulted another, who did operate. Because of her continued dissatisfaction with the results, and threats of suicide if he did not operate again, he performed several operations. When he finally refused to do any more, her agitation and vindictiveness grew. She sued for damages to her appearance, which by this time had been impaired, with the additional complaint that the operations had caused "traumatic psychoneurosis hysteria." She received a substantial settlement. Some months later a newspaper reported that she had been taken to a psychiatric hospital for attempted suicide.

THE POOR RISKS*

The Emotionally Disturbed

Not all forms of neurosis result from basic personality disturbances; some may be realistic responses to external situations. Yet, in the eyes of most surgeons, the fact that an individual has a

* See Notes at back of book.

record of emotional instability makes him immediately suspect, even when his complaint is valid. There is doubt whether surgery will satisfy him, whether he will become a management problem, or—worse still—whether surgery may precipitate a psychological collapse. His chances of being accepted are even less if he has the reputation of being hostile or a "personality problem."

John B., age 22, was such a person. When first seen by plastic surgeons in a Veterans Administration Hospital, where he had been admitted for a complaint diagnosed as psychosomatic, he was arrogant, defensive, and had untenable relationships with both personnel and patients. The surgeons described him as a "pain in the neck."

To a psychiatrist, J.B. had disclosed his feelings about his face and how it interfered with his relationships. He had what has been called the "FLK Syndrome" (funny-looking kid). His large ears stood out from the sides of his rather small head. His upper jaw protruded, making the teeth so prominent that he could not bring his lips together, and, in contrast, the lower jaw receded.

An otoplasty (surgery of the external ear) was permitted, but two surgeons discouraged additional surgery and orthodontic treatment lest these trigger a psychotic episode. In any event they regarded J.B. as "too difficult" and predicted he would be "a lot of trouble"—"I wouldn't touch him," said one—"He's a kook," said another. The psychiatrist didn't consider J.B.'s appearance significant in the etiology of his personality disorder and was skeptical about the psychological effectiveness of surgery. One resident surgeon, however, was inclined to operate. Because of conflicting opinions the patient was referred to the sociologist who was a member of the rehabilitation team.

A review of J.B.'s life history showed that his emotional problems had stemmed in large measure from ridicule and social rejection. At school his peculiar face on his small, thin body provoked the nicknames of "Long-legged Spider," "Elephant Ears," and "Buck Teeth"—epithets that he ruefully admitted were "appropriate—but this makes an impression. I always looked odd, and therefore I was considered odd."

Frequent family moves and new schools compounded his difficulties. Though bright, J.B. dropped out before finishing eighth grade.

You can't go to school if you're not accepted by the kids, and you can't learn something if everyone around you is making faces at you and you have arguments every morning. Kids are naturally going to pick on you. If you don't look right, you're singled out as the bad guy.

When he became interested in girls, his frustration continued. "I used to go up to a girl at a dance, but I was always rejected When I was young, everyone else went out with girls—I didn't." Convinced that he would have to go through life looking "odd," his efforts to cope with a hostile environment took the following forms:

He developed "a very short, sharp tongue." He rationalized leaving school on the grounds that he was "creative" and so musically gifted that he didn't need formal training, and, that since he was "talented," his looks weren't "the most important." To cover his real feelings of inferiority and insecurity he became arrogant and "put on an air of superiority and super-security." His isolation from others, he convinced himself, was self-imposed, since he had "superior intelligence and most other people were boring and unintelligent." Although his evaluation of his appearance was realistic, his defenses and coping stratagems only led to further social rejection, withdrawal, and more severe maladjustment.

J.B.'s growing intolerance of others multiplied his problems when he was drafted into the army. Hating it, he manifested symptoms such as shortness of breath and inability to perform routine physical activities. After hospitalization for bronchitis and pneumonia he refused to return to duty. Placed in a mental hospital, he was eventually given a psychiatric discharge.

His behavior at the VA hospital where he had undergone otoplasty tended to substantiate the surgeons' impressions of J.B.'s instability. His neurosis, however, was situational and his days were fraught with unmitigated humiliation. Surgery could not be expected to heal his psychic wounds, but correction of his appearance would remove a stigmatic barrier to his relations with others and help him to gain some self-esteem. For these reasons the sociologist endorsed surgery.

Postoperatively there was a striking change in J.B.'s face. Striking also was his dress: "mod" clothes, square gold-rimmed glasses, and ornate rings. He was delighted with the surgical results. He had begun to date and for the first time spoke hopefully of marriage. Although his improved appearance gave him an almost immediate sense of well-being and more confidence when meeting people, he had sufficient insight to realize that he lacked the skills of normal social interaction. "It will take a lot more time being with people to change from the way I was before. Because I kept to myself, I have to learn how to act around people. It's not that I'm not fairly well mannered and so on, but I can't carry on a conversation. There seem to be certain intricacies in human relationships that you have to learn before you can actually get along."

J.B. got a job as assistant nurse in a department of physical medicine. He found the patients interesting and enjoyed his work. Within a few months his former hostility and arrogance had almost vanished.

The Litigious

In a specialty that has one of the highest records for malpractice suits and consequently exceedingly high insurance rates, surgeons are perforce wary of accepting any candidate for surgery who they suspect may retaliate if his expectations are not fulfilled. Patients who have had cosmetic surgery elsewhere but wish additional operations tend to be viewed with caution. Blame, derogatory remarks about the original doctor, and vindictive attitudes are seen as red flags, and any hint of legal action is so threatening that most surgeons close the door on further considerations. The fear of suits for damages, realistic and justifiable as it may be in some cases, is so generalized that some patients who merit help are denied it. Caught in the rigid system of medical values along with the stigma attached to those who seek any form of retribution, such persons are left to work out their problems alone.

A case in point is that of S.F., who had a conspicuous pitting on her nose caused by a skin infection in her infancy, making her exceedingly self-conscious. At the age of 24 she consulted a plastic surgeon who performed dermabrasion[18] and rhinoplasty, which unfortunately resulted in further scarring and also notched alae (lower portion of side of nose). Four years later she requested evaluation at a plastic surgery clinic and was accepted for another dermabrasion. Dubious about this procedure because of its previous failure to eradicate the pitting, she asked instead for a skin overgraft. Although advised of the risk involved (possible scarring and difference in skin color), she chose to take the chance, preferring this possible outcome to the pitting. Moreover, she volunteered to sign any document exonerating the surgeons, should the operation fail.

While awaiting arrangement of her surgical appointment, S.F. mentioned to another patient that she had sued her first surgeon. The recipient of this information, an "old patient," told the head nurse. The surgeons' immediate reaction was to cancel the operation.

The story about the law suit was correct, but S.F. had not instigated it. Although she had been disappointed with the surgical results, so had the surgeon. Two days before operating he had broken his leg. According to S.F. he was in great pain and therefore hadn't done "as good a job as he might have. I felt sorry for him and I didn't blame him for what happened. He even offered to perform another operation." At the time S.F. was a secretary in a law firm. It was her employers who instituted procedures on her behalf, on the grounds that the surgery had been "botched up." She described the trial as "a terrible ordeal. I would never want to go through anything like it again." She still felt sorry for the surgeon and held no grudge. Her employers, however, had persisted and won the suit.

When the details of this case were reported to the surgeons who had refused to operate, S.F. was brought to the clinic conference for reevaluation. While several members of the group

18 Surgical removal of the outer layers of the skin to correct scars or wrinkles.

favored surgery, others more skeptical and worried about legal action vetoed the idea. The patient, whose hopes had been raised, left the clinic in tears.

The Persuaded*

Another poor risk for plastic surgery is the adult patient whose request for it has been brought about by pressure from other people rather than by his own inner needs. Regardless of the degree of the deformity, it may have certain value and meaning for the patient, and if so surgical correction may sometimes have an unforeseen and unwelcome effect.

Mr. J., a 58-year-old executive, had a marked facial paralysis acquired at age 6 as the result of an accident. Although his deformity was conspicuous, he had made a remarkable adjustment to it. Furthermore, he had achieved an enviable reputation in his profession and had recently been given a high position in a large insurance firm. His employer, who was struck by the obvious deformity, evaluated it in terms of his own attitudes toward physical deformities, that is, he felt that so noticeable an affliction was tragic and certainly handicapping. Eager to help, the employer called in a plastic surgeon to ascertain if an operation could improve the man's appearance. Upon being reasonably assured that it could, the employer informed Mr. J. that he and the surgeon wished to provide him with an opportunity to have his defect corrected. Mr. J. was touched by this gesture of thoughtfulness and generosity but found himself in an embarrassing position. He did not want an operation and had declined a similar suggestion by a surgeon some years before. All the same, he did not want to offend his employer or the surgeon by refusing their offer. He also began to wonder if holding his job depended on the correction of his deformity, which he now felt bothered his employer and by implication perhaps other personnel.

As a young boy he had been aware of the many disadvantages of having a facial paralysis, but he had compensated for it in many ways and had made adequate adjustments to it. His marriage was successful, and, because of his business acumen, every

* See Notes at back of book.

job was an advancement from the last. He had come to believe that his deformity was almost a mark of distinction. He even attributed to it much of his success: Because of it he had been driven to work harder and achieve some fame and in business no one ever forgot him.

Neither the employer nor the surgeon had provided him with the opportunity to discuss his feelings candidly, and Mr. J. felt obligated to agree to the operation. Nevertheless he was worried about what it would do to him psychologically. He was used to addressing large groups of people, but now he was afraid of being an object of curiosity and comment when he appeared before them again with what he called a normal face. He was also fearful that he would not get used to his new look and would become self-conscious.

Mr. J.'s situation had several serious aspects. First, he did not want an operation but was pressed by others to have one. Second, his deformity had been integrated in his total personality and had been used for secondary gains. Third, there were the risks inherent in any surgical procedure, such as possible infection or unforeseen complications, and, since the operation was not requested by the patient, any untoward event could conceivably have serious repercussions on the surgeon.

The operation was performed. No attempt was made to restore muscle activity but only to lift the sagging side of the face in order to achieve symmetry. There were complications. A mild infection occurred and the patient also developed pleurisy. Instead of the expected five days of hospitalization, Mr. J. remained for thirteen. The operation was not as successful as had been hoped, and no spectacular improvement was achieved. Six weeks later the patient had not returned to work, though he could have returned in two.

He had become exceedingly depressed and felt that he had gone through a prolonged ordeal for only a minor improvement. Although he had formerly dreaded returning to work with what he thought would be a startling new appearance, which would make him an object of curiosity, he now felt the situation to be more intolerable since those hearing about the operation would be disappointed in the results and feel sorry for him. All in all, the incident had served only to focus the attention both of the patient and his co-workers on the deformity. He had now become more self-conscious than he had ever been before. He felt himself helpless "for the first time in [his] life" and was questioning the advisability of returning to his job.

This case well illustrates the importance of not taking situations for granted, especially when the suggestion for surgery does not originate with the patient. Time should be given to careful interviewing of such a patient, no matter what the degree of the deformity, to understand what significance it may have for him.

In summary, the outlook is unfavorable if the patient reveals:

1. Confused, vague, and unconvincing explanations for requesting plastic surgery.
2. Motivation for surgery that is not a rational response to a realistic situation.
3. Excessive and unrealistic expectation of the results.
4. Dissatisfaction with previous plastic surgery operations.
5. A history of psychiatric disturbances.
6. Evidence that he places all responsibility for his difficulties in life on factors outside himself without insight into his own part in them.
7. The wish to eliminate a feature reminiscent of a rejected or rejecting parent.
8. Pressure from others to seek plastic surgery.

THE PYGMALION COMPLEX*

Although the plastic surgeon may sometimes be overly cautious in selection, he may also err on the side of suggesting surgery. For instance, his high sensitivity to the slightest deviation or asymmetry and his zeal to make "beautiful people" may tempt him to propose esthetic improvements. Referred to as the "Pygmalion Complex," this enthusiasm is a potential pitfall, one which can obscure the difference between the "desire to cure" and the "need to cure."[19] Surgeons' suggestions may also be motivated by pro-

---

* See Notes at back of book.

[19] Meyer, Eugene, "Psychiatric Aspects of Plastic Surgery," in *Reconstructive Plastic Surgery*, vol. 1, *General Principles*, edited by John M. Converse. W. B. Saunders Company, Philadelphia, 1964, pp. 365–383.

fessional self-interest, such as eagerness to obtain operating experience or to recruit patients—phenomena not uncommonly seen in resident training programs of teaching hospitals or in the building up of a practice.

While in some instances correction can safely be initiated and should be, the surgeon needs to be conscious of his motives. To suggest that an individual's appearance can be improved points up a deficiency and invites responsibility that must be carefully weighed. Should the person be unreceptive he will only be disconcerted. On the other hand, he may be more than ready to comply; but if he is dissatisfied with the outcome the doctor may have to bear the full onus.

Such a consequence was aborted in the case of R.L., age 39, who said she had come to the clinic because the previous week, while she was being treated for a sinus infection, a plastic surgery resident observed that rhinoplasty would make her look better. She asserted she had never thought of having an operation, but "since the doctor thought it would be a good idea" she was "willing" to have it.

Interviewing disclosed that R.L. actually had long desired to have her nose altered but had refrained for fear the result would fall short of her standards of perfection. In the event of an imperfect result she would have only herself to blame, a situation that she seemed psychologically unable to handle. Discussion of her work experience and social relationships revealed a need to hold others responsible whenever she failed. Fortuitously, in this instance, the resident's casual suggestion of a rhinoplasty had provided a solution to her dilemma. Should the operation fail to fulfill her hopes, he could be a convenient scapegoat.

CONFLICTING DEFINITIONS OF SUCCESS

Another source of problems in cosmetic surgery is the disparity between the surgeon's concept of a satisfactory result and the patient's expectations. Since the surgeon, by training, is necessarily concerned with reconstruction or correction that approximates in form and contour the anatomic "ideal"—nose, chin, ear, or breast —he assumes that the patient has the same image in mind. That there are cultural variations in concepts of the "ideal" may be forgotten. Confident in his judgment of what can and should be done, the surgeon is dismayed and puzzled when a patient is disappointed, although the results are technically successful.

Arbitrary ascription of physicians' standards in the controversial area of cosmetic surgery, where patients' responses are so often the criteria of "success," invites complications, as is shown in the following case:

Tired of being called "Ski Snoot" and teased about her "Bob Hope" nose, 29-year-old N.H. requested correction of its retroussé tip. The surgeon achieved what he considered an excellent result, but N.H. first wept hysterically, then became depressed. Though the modified tip pleased her, she had not expected the elimination of a slight dorsal concavity. To her this was a calamity because she was Irish and extremely proud of her heritage. Equating Irishness with a turned-up nose, she had tacitly valued the dorsal curvature. The surgeon's perception and creation of the "best" esthetic effect, in this instance a straight dorsum, destroyed what the patient prized—her Irish identity.

RELIANCE UPON OTHER PROFESSIONALS

Because of the exigencies of treatment, it is important for plastic surgeons to have other professionals on whom they can rely in making judgments in the patients' best interests. In most medical centers psychiatrists, clinical psychologists, and psychiatric social workers are available for referral and consultation, and it has become customary to turn to these specialists when questions arise regarding psychological diagnosis and management. They are also the ones most often included as participants in rehabilitation and research programs. Their use of such methods as interviews, psychological tests, and projective techniques often provides useful adjunctive information and insight in the team approach to comprehensive care.

In depending on these disciplines for psychosocial evaluations and solutions to behavioral problems, the plastic surgeon has also to be aware of certain limitations. The traditional training of psychiatrists, psychologists, and social workers is rooted in Freudian theory and individual psychology and, as such, focuses on personality development, the unconscious, and the intrapsychic processes of persons who manifest some form of psychopathology or behavior considered abnormal. This orientation, aimed at understanding the individual, is concerned primarily with such idiosyncratic features as his emotional life, personality structure, primary sexual identification, and the like. Interpretations of behavior considered deviant (which implies the existence of norms) tend to be couched in terms of pathology: repression, guilt, aggression, fixation, neurosis, and so on. Such interpretations fail to consider the person in the context of his social, cultural, and religious background, the influence of the social world in which he lives, and its impact on his attitudes and behavior.

Today the narrowness and shortcomings of the individual psychological approach to behavior are recognized, and there is increasing attention to broader perspectives that include those of sociology and anthropology. According to the noted psychiatrist Jurgen Reusch, emphasis must "shift away from man as an isolated entity and towards consideration of man in his environment."[20] His social needs must be considered, as well as his interdependence with his environment, including interaction with his surroundings. In similar vein Murphy states: "The conception of personality as a self-contained . . . whole . . . goes badly with the world of reality."[21]

For the person with cosmetic defects, his world of reality has unique import and must be taken into account. As already observed, his problems are frequently sociogenic rather than psychogenic. Referral to the psychiatrically oriented, therefore,

[20] Reusch, Jurgen, "The Future of Psychologically Oriented Psychiatry," in *Sexuality of Women*, edited by Jules H. Masserman, Grune & Stratton, New York, 1966, pp. 144–163.

[21] Murphy, Gardner, "Psychological Views of Personality and Contributions to Its Study," in *The Study of Personality: An Interdisciplinary Appraisal*, edited by E. Norbeck, D. Price-Williams, and W. M. McCord. Holt, Rinehart and Winston, New York, 1968, p. 33.

for diagnosis and solution of such patients' problems is not always the answer. Following are two cases in point.

Sarah was a 14-year-old girl whose lack of psychological readiness for surgery was the subject of a clinical conference. The surgeon suggested that the excessive anxiety of the mother was a factor in the child's resistance to a minor operation. The psychiatrist who had been called in to see Sarah declared that in his opinion the mother was not so much anxious as outright hostile toward her daughter—"What kind of mother was it," he asked, "who would slap her child's face on learning that the child's menses had begun?" This fact he had learned from Sarah herself while questioning her about the menarche. For him this was substantial and sufficient evidence of the mother's hostility, even cruelty. What he had failed to take into consideration, or to explore, was the possibility that there might be some other explanation.

Both Sarah and her mother were Orthodox Jews from East Europe, among whom it is the custom for the mother to slap her daughter's face at the time of the menarche "to bring roses to the cheeks," or to bring good luck. By assessing behavior in terms of his own cultural standards of the normal or abnormal, the psychiatrist was led to a false interpretation, for the mother's behavior was not aberrant. Because it was a custom of their culture, it had no deeper psychological implication for the child than the ritualistic and facetious spanking an American child is given on his birthday.[22]

C.A., a young mother of three, had incurred a slight facial scar in a car accident. In view of her low class and income level and her role as a housewife, her intense anxiety about her appearance seemed to the surgeons disproportionate and symptomatic of emotional disturbance. It was suggested that she needed a psychiatrist more than she did cosmetic surgery. C.A. happened to be Puerto Rican, and interviewing by the sociologist revealed that indeed

[22] Macgregor, Frances Cooke, *Social Science in Nursing: Applications for the Improvement of Patient Care.* Russell Sage Foundation, New York, 1960, pp. 23–24.

she had reason to be disturbed. In her sociocultural milieu a scar on a woman's face is a sign that one has been branded for unfaithfulness. She was distressed more for her husband, whom she loved, than about herself, since his acquaintances assumed he had slashed her cheek because she had had a lover. The stigma that Puerto Ricans attach to such scars was the sole reason both for her visit to the clinic and for what the surgeons had perceived as an "over-reaction." Fortunately in this instance a serious diagnostic error was averted.

CHAPTER EIGHT

Potential Lost and Potential Realized

POTENTIAL LOST

> The tragedy of life is what dies inside a man
> while he lives.
>
> (Albert Schweitzer)

THE CASE OF JANE LITTLETON

The victim of facial paralysis caused by damage to the facial nerve frequently finds that the ability to eat and speak with ease is impaired. Even worse, the ability to communicate by facial expression is destroyed: One eye may not close completely, an attempted smile turns into a grimace, and laughter becomes a mask of pain. Such was the plight of Jane Littleton. At age 2 her facial nerve had been accidentally damaged during a mastoid operation. Over the next twelve years a nerve graft and other treatments were attempted but without success.

In 1946, Jane, now 20, again sought help. In our initial interview she was defensive. Her eyes flashed angrily and her tone was defiant. It was apparent that any reference to her twisted face, which even in repose had a sardonic expression, was painful. Responses to questions were evasive and brusque. "No," her defect did not "bother" her; she had come to consult the surgeon at the urging of her co-workers at the post office where she had recently worked. "They told me I should have something done about my face, that I don't realize how bad it looks." Her last operation, performed a few years before, had failed. "It was my last hope." Though skeptical about improvement, she had heard that new surgical techniques were being developed and wondered if something might be done for her.

Currently, Jane was working in an artificial flower factory. For the past two years she and her only sibling, Roy (a truck driver, age 25), had been supporting their semi-invalid parents. Jane described her mother as a dominating and self-willed person whom she didn't like.

She keeps things stirred up with deliberate tongue lashings. When I'm mad I hit her. My father stays quiet. He has no will of his own. He's ugly. I can't take him anywhere. He's always dirty. He has a big nose and looks like a bad character. I feel ashamed when I'm with him. . . . My brother's changed since the war. He's quick-tempered, holds grudges, and argues a lot.

Although first directing her anger toward her family to the exclusion of her looks, Jane gradually revealed how much her distorted face distressed her.

I hold it against my mother. She probably let my ear infection go. People ask, "How did it happen?" Little children say, "Why don't you smile on the other side of your face?" And I have to say, "I don't know—I can't." When someone looks at me smiling and they look surprised, I stop . . . I notice people look over my shoulder when they talk. It makes me self-conscious—as though they didn't want to look at me. I'm embarrassed, so they think they're doing me a favor by looking over my shoulder. I'd rather have them look at me—back and forth—yet not stare. . . . It might be better to have it [surgery] done so I won't be shy.

To supplement the interview, Jane was asked if she would write an autobiographical sketch. She promptly produced several pages of memoirs, mainly in chronological sequence.[1] Although the extent to which imagination may have colored her recollections is a moot question, her perception of childhood experiences and reactions is eloquent in itself.

Background and Early Childhood

Jane's father, born in England, came alone to America some years after his marriage. Settling in an eastern city, and joined by his wife when their first child, Roy, was 3 years old, Mr. Littleton worked as a carpenter and later had his own car-wash business. According to Jane he provided adequately, but Mrs. Littleton "was always demanding more, and stirred up bitterness and strife." Two weeks after Jane's birth—Roy was then 5—their parents separated for what became an interval of eighteen years.

[1] The verbatim quotations in this case history have been excerpted and rearranged only as necessary to illustrate specific points.

The children lived with their mother until Jane's mastoid operation. During the three years that followed she was intermittently
hospitalized while a series of children's diseases "completed their
work of art."

During this time an auto accident crippled Mr. Littleton, and
he moved to a small house in the country where he could raise
chickens. Meanwhile, Mrs. Littleton had taken live-in laundress
jobs in institutions. As wards of a welfare agency, Jane and Roy
were virtually separated, too. Even when placed together in foster homes, the differences in their ages and interests, along with
Jane's frail health, precluded more than a tenuous bond.

> The Bonners [foster parents for six months] were very good and
> kind. They nursed me through a case of double pneumonia. I
> remember sitting in a blanket-lined wicker chair, on the sunny
> porch, eating peppermint candies.
>
> My brother and I didn't play together very much. He had other
> boys, while I sat on the steps and watched. There was nothing to
> do, and I would steal away to the main street, feeling very impor-
> tant walking in the crowds. My brother always was spanked for
> not watching me and complained he didn't see me leave.

The Disfigurement

Jane's next statement reports the first of a series of incidents
that display her awareness and sensitivity, and how she dealt with
the reactions of others to her appearance.

> [Age 4, at the Bonners.] One thing didn't please me—the camera.
> Though being very young, I understood its mechanism and its
> cause for existing. It grieved me to think anyone would want my
> picture. To be obliging and yet not completely so, I held my head
> downward.
>
> My brother had been teaching me to whistle, and one night after
> picking myself up off the floor and hopping into bed, I realized
> the first real whistle passed through my lips. This was really a
> great thing, because I thought whistling was impossible because
> my lips didn't come together straight.

> [Age 5, at a child care center.] The first day I stood by the door
> and cried. They noticed me, but that was all, and the children
> went right on playing with their toys. No one snickered or had
> any crocodile tears to spare.

[Ages 6–7, at another foster home.] This house had a beautiful garden, all the way from the back to the front. Every variety of flower and vegetable could be found. I enjoyed especially watching the goldfish among the water lilies in the pond. People stopped to look at the tulips, lily of the valley, and roses. I felt embarrassed while standing in front one day, but then I knew they were looking at the flowers and not at me.

One day while riding my bicycle through the path with some older school girls, they asked me if it hurt to laugh. When I said no, they were surprised.

On the school playground the children teased a colored girl. Against public opinion I stuck up for her, being very sure she was really white underneath. I never seemed to be the dunce of their play, but one time was a close shave. They gathered round me to look at the scratch the dog made on my nose. I feared someone would make another remark but they didn't, and I was so relieved.

[Age 7, at a childen's shelter.] Our school was a one-room affair, including all the classes. At promotion time the teacher said if I memorized a poem she would pass me. It was an old one that everybody knew except me. The big boy in front was gifted with leadership. They snickered over each line, making disgusting faces and altogether spoiling a lovely poem. It felt good to be in my seat again. I had a peculiar feeling because it was the first time I had ever stood in front of them without running away. It seemed I had conquered.

The Other Side of the Coin

Although Jane's recollections of her fifteen years in hospitals, shelters, foster homes, and boarding schools reflect her insecurity, they nevertheless emphasize positive relationships and experiences. The following passages typify her interests, observations, and attitudes.

[Age 5.] It was good to be in the Children's Aid. There were swings, a tent, toys, and a lady who told us stories, besides lots of good food. I remember having a nice girlfriend. We played in the tent and took turns on the swings. She showed me how much fun it was to push the little ones.

One day while I was sitting in a high chair eating some good hot oatmeal, a lady who had been looking at me said, "Now, Janie, this is the way to hold your spoon." Someone else came and having different opinions held their spoons right in front of each other's nose. . . . Finally the first one admitted she was wrong and peace was once again restored. It seemed strange to be the cause of an argument but not in any way be involved.

[Ages 6–7.] Betsy [child of foster parents] and I had many good times together. We baked mudcakes on the old car, played house, looked for good stones on the driveway, and made doll clothes. Her mother kept us supplied with cookies, scissors, and material. Whenever there was a dispute about possessions, Betsy took them back again. The little tyke was younger, but when she had the ideas first, what could I say?

[Age 7, in the hospital.] There was a boy with two broken legs that were stretched straight up in the air. He had a way that said "I'm your friend." He loaned me his clay when I first came. But there were others who were mean and mimicked me. I'd try to get a friend and she'd go with someone else.

When Nancy came, things began to change. Her face, chest, and arms were badly burned and her lips couldn't close. Her speech was hindered and she dribbled constantly. She had dark, short, straight hair, with unusually big eyes. But her happy disposition brightened the whole ward. During those days we did most things together. We ate our meals in the kitchen and helped dry dishes, while the others had rest hour. We played with the baby on the sun porch and made tents of blankets and sheets with the extra beds there. Sometimes we would start to play school, and wind up drawing pictures on the slates.

[Age 7, at a shelter.] Haverford House is an institution that examines children before they are admitted to other schools. This period may be from three to six months long. I remember sneaking down to eat some of my candy, and while admiring the lawns and shrubbery, the thought occurred to me that it's not the looks of the building, but the people in it that count. Their attitude toward each other makes for happiness or discontent.

At night a lady came and gave us cookies. We really enjoyed them and tried to see who could keep theirs the longest. When the lights were out, some of us, including me, hopped out of bed and crawled under the others thinking we frightened them. We did this every night and never tired.

[Ages 7–14, at a boarding school.] In the summer time of 1933 I caught my first glimpse of the Delaware River, shimmering under the afternoon sun. Its peaceful quietness and the dignity of air [sic] spoke of a different rhythm of life. Something good and greatly to be desired. Even the trees knew it, and the car as it sped along the road. When I arrived at St. Paul's I found the children of Green Cottage were fun.[2] They were taking baths upstairs, and Mrs. Vance made Mary laugh while she was in the tub. Irene Barnes loaned me her doll. We played tag that night and somehow I was it too often. Joyce Johnson, a chubby little redhead, was the baby. She was cute, with laughing big blue eyes. Amy Bennett could run very fast.

During those days someone was always teaching me something. Christine, the school teacher, taught me the books of the Bible; Marie, with patient manner, table manners; Ellen, how to make a neat bed; and Gwen, to be the first one up on those cold mornings when the bell rang.

The piano was a very popular instrument with everyone. We would often rush into the room to see who could get it first. There were many good books too. Sometimes we would read one constantly for two or three days to finish it.

Each one of us, even tomboy Gwen, liked to be always neat. Our bureau drawers, lockers, and beds were immaculately neat, with Amy's the best and Donna's a close second. I soon learned sloppy stockings and muddy shoes didn't belong here.

We were always busy. In the winter we went sleigh riding on the hill or raced each other out to the summer house, while the wind blew us inside out. During the summer we enjoyed diving into the shallow pool, swinging on the swings, or going on long hikes with Miss Goetz. There were extra things, like trips to the city or having a magician visit us.

The large sitting room was the scene of many parties and nutcracking in front of the fireplace. During the mornings, especially Saturdays, it seemed the radio and magazines interferred [sic] with its cleaning speed. An older girl always had the room and kept the door closed long enough for us to lose our tempers. During Christmas there was a huge tree in the corner. We always enjoyed the holidays and regretted going home.

When the new gym was built we started playing basketball games with other schools. One year as we had our banquet Gwen and I were awarded medals. Trudy Reed really deserved it, and I felt badly for taking it. Trudy, besides being beautiful, had developed natural abilities that made her very special. She was full of ideas, from making doll clothes to play acting.

In this atmosphere all thought of being inferior or ashamed was gone. I felt happy and free to act without criticism. When Mrs.

---

[2] Before Jane's arrival at the School, a perceptive head mistress had prepared the other children for Jane's deformity. Their acceptance of her and her contented years there were no doubt due in great measure to the sensitive management of her handicap.

Vance hinted something would be tried to help my face, I was surprised they were interested in that too and felt I couldn't appreciate all their kindness. Later, after Dr. X's operation, it was necessary to have electric treatments in town three times a week. The trainman knew me so well he would hold the train as I came running down the steps from the other side.

High School Years

Because the age limit for residence at St. Paul's was 16, Jane had to leave two years before completing high school.

Then one day I said goodbye to all my friends and moved to the unbeautiful part of the suburbs known as "the sticks." Here I lived with my father in a tiny three-roomed house.[3] This section of Hopedale only boasted a firehouse and two stores. All my happiness would have disolved [sic] if it were not for a good friend, my neighbor. She had a soft way about her that made everyone welcome at her house, and we . . . spent many happy hours together.

Apparently Jane took in stride the transition to a public high school but her report, while emphasizing the satisfactory aspect, is cursory.

The Alma Mater of Ricks High School is only a part of its beauty. The sweet hum of busy children and the quietness during exams contrasts with the happiness but yet the solemn seriousness of four years of work. The charm and natural loveliness of a country school keeps its beauty in modern design, giving it a dignified air. There are things about the school that become a part of every student. If it isn't the huge field, working on the school paper, sweating in the gym or at their locker, then they [sic] tell you of their wrestling record or the fun they had in a play. The art, typing, shop or homemaking rooms were never idle.

Everyone liked Ricks! Before the bell rang students stood around their lockers in the hall, talking. It was easier to walk with someone rather than alone. In my second year I gained a little in popularity and fame. By staying after school for sports I made lots of friends.

[3] Jane's mother still lived and worked in an institution but had begun to spend weekends at home and helped out financially. Two years later, incapacitated by an accident, she came home to stay and never worked again.

In an interview Jane also had mentioned her "many friends" found in athletics and in the girls' glee club. She had never dated, however, and regretted missing the school dances. She thought she "didn't have the ability to talk with boys," felt inadequate, and "wondered how other girls did it." She claimed to "like pretty girls—not envy them" and "watched the way they dressed and what they said."

Jane's recollections gloss over her deformity and paint a picture of acceptance and adjustment to it. Her rapid embracing of religion, however, would indicate her need of support.

The Presbyterian Church had a large number of children in its Sunday School. This man teacher seemed to put a lot in his lessons and yet it is effortless. What was he saying? "Ye must be born again?" I never heard that before. My! how beautiful he speaks of Jesus. What a great treasure the Bible is!

One day I went to Mrs. Maxwell's house to help her with her new baby. When she was well again I went to her Bible Class. Later we had prayer meetings together, and they started a Sunday School in their basement. During prayer one night I accepted the Lord as my Savior. By His grace on the cross I knew my sins were forgiven, and I love my Savior who gave His life for me. His Blood was shed that you and I might spend eternity at His, our Savior's side.

Jane's high school reminiscences concluded as follows:

I graduated in June 1944 [age 18]. The armed service had taken some of our would-be graduates. The "mighty" Max with his butch haircut and German march. There were others too, but eloquent Tim Mooney was with us to deliver a stirring message of the good times of Ricks and the challenges ahead.

Vocational Fumbling

Information on Jane's intellectual ability was scant. Her public high school major in home economics "bored" her; she had wanted to become a physical education teacher. She said she was not permitted to take college entrance examinations, however, because her "aptitude tests showed no material." (See page 192 for a later and contradictory evaluation.) Her earlier investigation of nursing as a possible career had been discouraged by a nurse who believed the sight of Jane "might cause someone a nervous breakdown or relapse. . . . [She] advised me that nurses with defects have a bad psychological effect on patients, who, being ill, may think, 'If she can't help herself, how can she help me?' "

With both parents unemployed, Jane felt obliged to take whatever work she could get. Directly from high school she obtained a job in a laundry but soon left "because the work was too hard." Next she sorted mail in a post office but was "laid off." It was here that plastic surgery had been suggested to her. Although currently working in the artificial flower factory, she was anxious to continue her education and was taking geometry at night school. She described her life as "getting up, working, and going home." She had no friends among the girls in the factory. "They gossip and I get hurt easily." Her only social outlet was going to church, where she also taught a Sunday School class. She once remarked, "I think I would like to be married. If it comes, it comes." Then, as if to acknowledge the improbability of it, she added with vehemence, "But it's not the only thing in the world!"

The Operation

In 1947 Jane underwent surgery designed to support her sagging facial muscles by means of a fascial sling, a procedure performed inside the cheek. Although it does not restore muscle control, it may effect some symmetry of the face in repose. In Jane's case improvement was minimal.

The Denouement

Nothing more was heard from or about Jane until 1967. Then from a distant state mental hospital where she was a patient, she wrote Dr. Y at the plastic surgery clinic requesting an appointment. She complained of a tightness in her mouth which interfered with the wearing of dentures. The name, "Jane Littleton," roused no recollection of her case nor could any records be located. Nevertheless a letter was sent to the state hospital director suggesting Jane come to the clinic. There was no reply.

Eight months later Jane again wrote to Dr. Y stating that to obtain permission to travel to the clinic she had to have an escort. More delay ensued because neither state hospital nor clinic could provide such services. At this impasse, a third letter from Jane came, by chance, to the attention of the sociologist who had first interviewed her and who, recognizing her name, immediately contacted Dr. Z, Jane's psychiatrist at the state hospital. Dr. Z, pleased to learn that Jane could be seen by her former surgeon, offered full cooperation. "Jane never belonged here in the first place," she said, "and anything that might lead to her discharge is of great importance."

What had happened to Jane since we last saw her? Following her last operation she had continued to live with and support her parents until her father's death several years later and her mother's admission to a rest home. Her brother meanwhile had married. Jane, now in her early thirties, inherited the little house. No longer working, and friendless, she remained in virtual seclusion with a collection of stray dogs on which she showered affection. As new homes grew up around her, the occupants complained that Jane's dwelling was a health hazard because it lacked plumbing and her unlicensed dogs were kept indoors. Financially unable to comply with the orders of the authorities and refusing to relinquish her "only friends," she was sentenced to several days in jail and eventually committed by court order to the state hospital where she became ID #647267A. While she was confined there her property was condemned and sold.

Separation from her home and her pets was a severe blow. On hospital admission at the age of 33, Jane was found "untidy, withdrawn, and negativistic; showed slight depression and some emotional dulling; and her insight and judgment were poor." Her memory and sensorium were intact, however.

Her IQ test showed her to be high average, and her intellectual potential superior. At the same time she was considered "severely retarded emotionally and functioning more as a child than as an adult." Her high school report at the time of her graduation described her behavior as normal. "She was kind hearted, good-natured, and tried to please everyone. However, she had developed an inferiority complex because of her appearance."

After some three years of "changeable" behavior in the hospital, "sometimes more, sometimes less cooperative," Jane was placed on ground parole but took no advantage of it, electing only to spend her free time on the hospital grounds feeding the birds and stray cats. Though all along her psychiatric tests had been diagnostically negative, she remained in the institution for want of a place to go. Attempts by her custodians to find a home where she could baby-sit had failed because of her disfigurement and the possibility of its "frightening the children."

Dr. Z described Jane as having become friendly, thoughtful, and compliant.

> She helps us here in the treatment rooms and doing things for us. She's so willing and such a nice girl, and so appreciative of any kindness shown her. She's slightly retarded socially—not mentally. She is shy and has an inferiority complex because of her appearance. . . . She is now allowed to go alone to visit her mother in the nursing home. Apparently she gets along very well with her mother, and they seem to be very attached to each other. . . . She doesn't belong here and could be discharged immediately if she had a place to go.

Soon after Jane started visiting the nursing home, the director suggested that she live there and help care for her ailing mother. Since this arrangement would enable her to have escorted visits to the clinic, Jane was discharged—after ten years of hospitalization.

The Clinic Revisited

A month later Jane came to the clinic. We had not seen her for twenty-three years. She sat hunched in a corner of the reception room, looking older than her 43 years. Her institutional clothes were shabby and ill-fitting: an old-fashioned coat, rumpled blouse, and someone's cast-off taffeta evening skirt. Incongruous and childlike were her white bobby socks, shoes she had decorated with gold braid, and the yellow gift-package ribbon around her hair. When she first talked to me, she raised her eyes rather than her head. She looked beaten, though her eyes sparkled at times when something humorous was said. Where once she created the impression of wearing a chip on her shoulder and of being quick to anger, making snappy answers to questions, she now lacked affect and appeared resigned. There seemed little fight left in her.

With no trace of bitterness Jane recounted the events of the long interval during which we had not seen her. The period following her last operation had been very trying—"Instead of my face being beautiful and lovely to look at, it was just the opposite. I didn't attract very much attention, as I kept pretty much to myself, so I didn't hear anybody's unintentional remarks or queer expressions concerning my appearance."

She had believed she could always go on living where she was—"in my simple beautiful place, but I soon found out that it couldn't be done. I had no money for a lawyer and the judge sent me to the state hospital. I didn't want to go and I was very frightened; I thought people would be much sicker than they are." In time Jane became interested in the handicrafts offered as occupational therapy and she liked working in the treatment room. Although she wanted to leave, she had no choice.

I couldn't sign out. I didn't know the rules of the hospital. We are on the ward. [Note transition to present tense, as if being "out" were still not quite real to her.] We don't see anybody. There are no rule books. There are two or three attendants on the ward, but they're very busy, and you have to have someone with authority to tell you what you can do.

There are some 10 to 15 thousand patients . . . and if each doctor had to talk to each patient it would be impossible. All you know is what you hear from other patients. If the doctors would only have a meeting with 50 or 100 patients so we could ask questions—but they don't, and it's difficult for them to know all about us. They're not there all the time. It's difficult to get the records, and also notes are left about patients and sometimes they're exaggerated or not true. I didn't bother Dr. Z [her psychiatrist] as I had no place to go.

There is no communication system there like we had in school, where they would ring a bell and inform students over the radio. They just put patients in a room; they eat and sleep well, and that's all.

A lot of people there have queer ideas in their heads, and they find it is a snug place to live. If their records are too good, they'll deliberately do something so they won't be sent out. Most of them are afraid of autos and having sudden accidents.[4]

[4] This seemed to be true of Jane also who frequently reminded the interviewer that it was dangerous to fly and one should be able to stay near home.

Plastic Surgery Reconsidered

Although Jane's present complaint concerned a functional impairment, the examining surgeons also addressed themselves to the esthetic improvements that advanced techniques could now provide. Recommended was a lifting of her right cheek to achieve symmetry, excision of the overhanging upper lip, and a prosthesis that would enable her to close her left eye. To the doctors' surprise Jane declined all surgery except the remedial procedure for which she had come. "Yes," she told us, "once I was interested in having my appearance corrected. I was younger then, but I am a lot older now. Since the face is not a matter of life or death, it's not so important. I think that once you take care of a medical problem that is sufficient." Then, as if seeking approval of her decision she added, "There are a lot of other problems in the world, don't you think?"

Although she was deeply grateful to the clinic personnel for their interest and especially for effecting her release from the hospital—"I would have stayed there *forever!*"—Jane's concern about her appearance had obviously faded. During her years at the mental institution, among inmates and staff, her deviant appearance was inconsequential. Moreover it was not the barrier to satisfying human contacts it had been in the world outside.

Now Jane is in another protective environment, a community of those handicapped by age who both accept and need her. Though with some wistfulness she says she wishes she could work on the "outside" and earn some money, the idea of correcting her appearance to make this possible is threatening. Her disability has in actuality become her security. She is content where she is. She is "happy" to be helping her mother, it is pretty in the country, and she has kittens to play with. In sum, she regards herself as fortunate because "so many people have been so kind to me and," as she added resignedly, "much of the time just goes away."

POTENTIAL REALIZED

THE CASE OF NATALIE LUBIN

When Natalie Lubin at 18 was seen at the Plastic Surgery Clinic, the staff at first sight judged her to be mentally retarded. Born with a craniofacial anomaly known as Apert's Syndrome she had multiple deformities: bulging wide-set eyes that focused unevenly; a lumpy, shapeless nose; flattened mid-face bones; and a half-open, carp-like mouth. Additional handicaps associated with her condition were the stumpy hands, whose short fused fingers had been separated in infancy, and her fused toes, still uncorrected. Compounding her esthetic problems was an unsightly case of acne.

Natalie was accompanied by her mother, an intelligent but harried, chain-smoking woman whose demeanor with the social worker had immediately earned her the labels "difficult" and "hostile." By contrast Natalie was friendly, outgoing, and anxious to please. Though her speech was often blurred, her animated and rapid-fire responses came as a surprise to those meeting her for the first time, but no more so than the information that she was in high school and hoped someday to be a teacher!

Natalie was born in New York City and lived there in a middle-class housing project. She was the first child of second-generation Russian Jewish parents. She had a sister two years younger. When Natalie was 12, her father, an insurance salesman, died following a long illness. To supplement their seriously depleted income Mrs. Lubin worked part time as an assistant bookkeeper and receptionist in a doctor's office.

Following the birth of their defective baby, the grieving parents in conference with the doctors were faced with an agonizing decision. Although it was too early for definite diagnosis, the doctors were concerned about possible brain damage and/or mental retardation, and they suggested alternative courses of action to the parents: Give the baby away, leave her in the hospital for a year for observation, or take her home. One physician said, "If it were my child and I gave her away, or left her in the hospital and at the end of a year found there was a chance she was normal, I'd never forgive myself."

So Natalie was taken home. But for months the parents were in deep despair, a despair intensified by the marital strain precipitated by Mr. Lubin's claim that Mrs. Lubin was somehow responsible for their tragedy. Mr. Lubin, described by his wife as a handsome and practical man who had never had a sick day in his life, was "overwhelmed" by the fact of his defective child. "He couldn't face it—he stopped sleeping and he stopped working—he just fell apart." When he began to "agonize" about the impending financial strain with respect to Natalie's care and her future, Mrs. Lubin accused him of feeling more sorry for himself and of being unable to face the fact that his child wasn't born "perfect." In desperation she told him, "If you feel sorry for the child, get a different job. Go out and make even more money if you think that money will help. But if you feel sorry for yourself then please leave us alone. Go wherever it makes you happy; go with the beautiful people!" Meanwhile Mrs. Lubin, in a semishocked state, remained secluded at home. "I didn't go out on the street for six months. I mean no make-up, no getting dressed. Finally we started to pick ourselves up. My husband took a new job with his cousins and I got dressed and we went about our business. But I'm not going to tell you it's easy to face the world."

Neurological examinations when Natalie was a year old revealed no brain damage. The tendency she had to carry her head to one side was remedied by an operation on an eye muscle, but because of potential complications the parents were told that attempts at facial reconstruction might cost the child her life, and nothing more was done at the time to improve her appearance.

Six months later Natalie's parents consulted a plastic surgeon about her hands and feet. Mrs. Lubin said:

There I was, sitting and crying like a waterfall. And the doctor said, "Why are you crying? You *have no right to cry*," and he came back with some pictures of a baby boy. (You know that story? "I cried because I had no shoes, so I met a man who had no feet"—that's only from the books.) I had never seen webbed hands until Natalie was born. I had never seen that you could be born with stumps from the wrist up: So he showed me the pictures. He said, "Now look, you see this picture of this little boy? He has no hands. If *that* mother cries I can understand it. I can't give that child hands. But your child has hands. I will separate the fingers." Returning home I told my sister, "I am the luckiest woman in the world. I saw pictures of a child born without hands and my child has hands."

A series of four operations was required to separate Natalie's fingers. But the surgeon thought it inadvisable to operate on her feet. Mrs. Lubin recalled:

He told us, "If she walks let her alone. If you can spare this child any tears, even the normal crying that it is sometimes necessary to make the child go through for her own good, *spare* her. She's gone through such hell." And we went home—when my husband said, "You know, the doctor is such a fine person that he would love to spare this child any tears, but I'm not going to listen to him." And I said, "Why?" He said, "Well, someday when we're gone the world is not going to coddle her, so I'm going to be very strict and make her toe the mark, so that by comparison the world will be almost kind." And as a result he was very, very strict with her. And she loved him deeply—more so than she does me, if that's possible, because she is basically a loving child. I think you don't have to teach a child to feel love. If he's sheltered, he feels it automatically. What's good for a child is good for a child whether he's the most beautiful or the most handicapped. There's no rules. What we want is to be *equal*, whether we're black, white, Jew, Gentile, anything. And I think what we want when we have handicaps—I don't think anyone is born perfect— we want to be treated *equal*, not necessarily better. It's when we're treated worse that it appears we're striking out, we want even better. But no, equal is good enough. And it was fortunate that my husband got the idea *not* to give her the sympathy and extra attention because it wouldn't be constructive. So he said, "I'll treat her as if she was perfect, because if she's my child I love her. But if I'm going to feel sorry for her then I may hurt her—so if I want to give her any kind of legacy to face this world, I've got to prepare her for it. And coddling is no preparation."

Shortly after Natalie was born, Mrs. Lubin decided to have another child. She said, "I had to do that for my own mind.[5] I said to myself, 'If I have another child and it's all right Natalie will have a sister or brother'—which was terribly important— 'and if, God forbid, the next child isn't born perfect, well, I *had* it already.' And I was ready. It was false courage, but I had to

---

[5] Though she did not say so, it is more than likely that she hoped to prove to her husband that she could have a normal child.

gamble. And so when this other child came out perfect I was happy." Meanwhile the parents resumed their desperate search for a plastic surgeon who would try to make Natalie's face presentable, but were repeatedly turned down. "What is this child going to do when she understands *why* people are staring at her?", Mrs. Lubin asked herself, for Natalie had become aware of being stared at. She told me:

> You'll find that laymen stare in a more studying fashion than a doctor or nurse. I used to say to Natalie, when someone stared at her unnecessarily and too long and she would sort of be uncomfortable—I used to say, if I felt nasty or weak, "That's all right Natalie, this is a doctor or a nurse, and they must *study* you!"

Because Natalie was too young to understand the word "normal," her mother tried to explain that some children are born with a long nose, others with a short nose, some with blue eyes and some with green, and so on. She said:

> I told her, for [my] lack of formal training, that if she will be good —you know, good—kind and loving, she will become beautiful. And when you're very, very young, you believe your mother. You don't think for yourself. And I felt that would suffice at that tender age, and I was hopeful that when she grew up she would know the beauty I mean, which came from within. Because when I was a child, to me the most beautiful woman in the world was Eleanor Roosevelt—because when she started a speech she was just beautiful and that's where I got that premise [sic] I'm sure— my reaction to Eleanor Roosevelt.

About Natalie's hands, Mrs. Lubin told her:

> If you ever feel bad that your hands don't look as perfect as the next child, remember that when I took you to Dr. B. the first time when you were a very little baby, he showed me how lucky we are. He showed me a picture of a little boy who had been born without hands. Now, is it *terrible* that your hands aren't like the next one's? Can't you do everything with your hands?

Because Natalie was quick to learn—she could sing, dance, and swim—her mother sent her to public school so that she might have as "normal" a childhood as possible. "But you will never know what that child went through," Mrs. Lubin said, "and never did she cry or complain." The children taunted her, and some days she would come home with her hair stuck together with chewing gum. There were teachers, too, who were repelled by her gargoyle-like face and, because it tended to invalidate assumptions of learning ability, gave her scant attention. The occasional one who did, however, would earn Natalie's "undying devotion." To keep her going, Mrs. Lubin provided her with special tutoring until it was discovered that Natalie could do as well as the other children, but Natalie dissipated all her energies in "looking for someone to like her." Ostracized as she was, she spent her time after school on the block where she was known, talking to older people, running their errands, and offering to watch their small children, a pastime in which she found her greatest joy.

When Natalie was 12 years old, Mr. Lubin died. He had been ill for five years with heart disease, a condition Mrs. Lubin believed was directly related to his "worries and aggravations over Natalie and finances."

All along Natalie's relationship with her sister, Sylvia, had been one of constant conflict and quarreling. At an early age Sylvia, who was pretty and very bright, voiced her concern about Natalie's "differentness" and asked her mother if Natalie would ever look the same as other people when she grew up. Sylvia had many friends but was ashamed of Natalie and excluded her from all their activities. Even when Sylvia herself became obese, a condition attributed both to her feelings about Natalie and to the loss of her father to whom she was closest, she persisted in rejecting Natalie.

During these years Mrs. Lubin struggled constantly to bolster Natalie, to give her faith in herself, and to encourage her independence. She also made a point of treating Natalie and Sylvia as "equals." Said Mrs. Lubin: "As far as I was concerned, the two girls are equal. I kept telling Natalie and hoping she would believe me and hoping I would believe myself as I heard it, 'There isn't anything you can't do in this world if you want to badly enough. Anything can be accomplished.' "

Both Mrs. Lubin and Natalie thought it would be "the most wonderful thing in the world" if Natalie could be a nursery school teacher. "Natalie is so wonderful with little children," her mother said. "You don't know how she babysits for a child; with *such love*." Women who had watched Natalie in the park with youngsters told Mrs. Lubin that they had never seen anyone treat children as she did. Mrs. Lubin recognized, however, that if Natalie did not fulfill the academic requirements she could not realize her aim. She was worried because Natalie was so anxious to be accepted that she didn't concentrate. She needed to be more motivated "because work will save her life."

By the time Natalie was 18 she had managed to get as far as the twelfth grade—her promotions had been largely "charitable"—but she could not apply herself. She was so inattentive and hyperactive that her class performance was "abominable," according to the principal, and did not even reflect that of "a kid in the low normal mental range." She seemed headed for failure. The principal considered Natalie's and her mother's goals, an academic diploma and teaching little children, completely unrealistic.

At that time Mrs. Lubin read an article about the successful reconstructive work of a plastic surgery unit at a nearby medical center, and she quickly made an appointment. The peculiar problems involved in creating an esthetically acceptable face for Natalie seemed insurmountable, and the consensus of all but the chief surgeon was that hers was a "hopeless case." Not too certain himself of how much, if any, improvement could be achieved, he nevertheless initiated plans for treatment. Beginning with correction of the protrusion of Natalie's eyes, there would be a series of operations to be spread over a period of years, and which, at this writing six years later, is not yet completed. Natalie and her mother viewed her acceptance by the surgeon as a "miracle," and Natalie could hardly wait for surgery to begin. Any absences from school, however, would undoubtedly end her chances for graduation. To forestall this required the coordinated efforts of the hospital social worker, the school, and the vocational rehabilitation agency enlisted to fund her education. Arrangements were made for Natalie to be tutored at home for a year during which she would repeat the twelfth grade and, it was hoped, graduate. But this accomplishment was not without its problems: The first teacher refused the assignment because he saw his pupil as a "fetus," nor did the high school principal initially approve, because he believed that pursuing a course toward an academic diploma was not in Natalie's best interest.

Natalie invariably expressed delight with the results of each surgical procedure. Though her face might be discolored and swollen, her deep emotional need for the promised effects led her to see dramatic improvement where others saw very little. Despite the pain and discomfort, occasional setbacks and infections, she never complained. Even following an 8-hour operation, with half her scalp shaved and her face still distorted from the after effects, she was enthusiastic. "Dr. K. is fantastic. Anything he does is marvelous."

As gradual changes were made on her face (they were mainly reductions in the extent of the deformity), coupled with the attention and positive reinforcement she received from those interested in her rehabilitation, Natalie's studies improved and at the end of a year she received her high school diploma. Now her optimism about the future was high, and she wanted to get a college degree and teach handicapped children "to show them how they can live a normal life like me." But her grades were too low and on the advice of her vocational counselors she was enrolled in a school for the handicapped where her suitability for college, or for a less demanding vocational program, could be determined.

Of interest to those working with Natalie at this time were her ability to maintain her psychological equilibrium and, despite her lamentable imperfections, her vigilant efforts to present a social mask of a "normal" young woman. By denying the reality of her situation—an "*as if* it doesn't exist" method sometimes employed by markedly disfigured persons who endeavor to function socially—she was able to cope. As seen by her responses to a Sentence Completion Test, she had internalized much of her mother's exhortation:

1. *My face*—is not important to boys or anyone, it's my personality. If I'm supposed to have something, I will get it regardless of my face.
2. *I suffer*—hardly ever, there is no need to.

3. *My nose*—is only there for smelling, and does not tell anything about me.
4. *I fear*—nothing.
5. *My greatest trouble*—there is really no trouble.
6. *My eyes*—are blue.
7. *I envy*—no one. Why should I? I can do anything I want if I put my mind to it.
8. *The future*—can only be what you make it.
9. *My lot in life*—is to succeed.
10. *My dreams*—can be fulfilled if I try.

On a deeper level, however, Natalie was far from secure. Psychological tests revealed an underlying depression as well as guilt feelings for "having been born this way." They also showed that although Natalie's basic intellectual endowment was close to bright normal, "performance function" was depleted by her anxiety and her feelings of self-depreciation about her body image.

Despite her underlying depression, the tester felt that Natalie's overt spontaneity and motivation to help herself were strengths which should not be lost sight of. In sum, Natalie was well aware of the magnitude of her problem, but continued to hope and work toward a more independent life and was making "gargantuan efforts to adjust and cope."

In the accepting environment of the school for the handicapped, where the social reality of her impediment was less abrasive, Natalie continued to make progress despite ongoing medical treatment, and at the end of a year she was allowed, under a special aids program, to enroll at a nearby college. On trial, she was to take two courses. She was then 21.

In her new surroundings, Natalie felt herself an outsider. Instead of studying she retreated to her babysitting "not for the money, but because the children love me. I love them, I spoil them rotten." Lacking friends her own age she had attached herself to a neighbor's son five years younger than herself and for the first time had a companion with whom to window shop, ride subways, and go to movies. While Mrs. Lubin regarded such a relationship "inadvisable under normal circumstances, in Natalie's case it was therapy, it was better than the clinic." But as Natalie's attachment to Marvin grew Mrs. Lubin worried lest there be in Natalie's fantasies more than a platonic relationship. She also recognized the potential hurt for Natalie when Marvin would find other friends (as of course he did). Warning her daughter of this eventuality, she stressed again the necessity of study, of "having work or a career to find pleasure in—so if your one friend goes away, it won't be so *terrible*."

Although Mrs. Lubin was proud of Natalie's ability to ignore "with dignity" the reactions and rebuffs of others, to go about her affairs, and at the same time to "be so friendly and loving," she had many misgivings. She wondered if she had done the right thing by telling Natalie that she was "equal." Recently Natalie wanted to answer an advertisement for a job for which she would "obviously" be unacceptable. On another occasion she had suggested that her mother "find a nice man and get married," saying "Daddy's never going to come back, and in a few years if Sylvia and I get married you will be alone." Mrs. Lubin said she had been criticized by relatives and friends for Natalie's "unrealistic" notions about the future and for allowing her to go through life thinking she was just like others. "They say, 'It wasn't fair to put her here—and you put yourself in a dream world too; she's not equal, she doesn't *look* the same.' Sometimes I say bitterly, sometimes facetiously, 'I don't think she's equal, no, I think she's *better*.'"

In all our interviews Mrs. Lubin expressed feelings of inadequacy, self-denigration, guilt, and resentment. Her lack of education—she wished she could have gone to college and become a doctor or a nurse—had left her "unprepared for a situation of this kind. I'm just a mother; what I do for Natalie any cleaning woman can do—I mean—you know, clothing and things like that. . . . Natalie is more than a child, she's a *project*!"

Mrs. Lubin was aware that although Natalie apparently welcomed each arrangement for another surgical procedure, her anxiety manifested itself in emotional turmoil and exacerbation of her acne.

You can't imagine what suffering this child has gone through medically and emotionally because of the problems she has. Sometimes when she is sitting alone, I can see she's reflecting and thinking of what she's gone through or something. The expression is sad—when you always see her ready to laugh and be bubbly. What does she say? I don't even like to think of it (tearfully). Sometimes I say, "What are you thinking about?" I just make it an offhand question. "You look so serious." Sometimes she says, "I think a lot of kids don't realize how lucky they are. What if they hadda go through what I hadda go through?" Or, "Suppose Dr. K. can't help me," or whatever.

Then you have the social suffering of not being accepted by children of your own age—children are cruel because they're innocent or ignorant. Then you have ignorant adults who can hurt you more than innocent children. Then, the tests, the x-rays, the interviews —emotionally and physically—all these things which you don't even talk about. You just talk about specifics—operations. Do you realize how much emotion goes in when you just go to the doctor's office? Like the last visit we had. Natalie sits there while Dr. K. and Dr. M. talk about what they hope to do and everything. You see the color in her face change. Such a tense moment. It's a moment of happiness—maybe—"that it'll help me"—fear of the pain—fear of not going to school—or falling further behind. And I watch her facial expressions. And she sits there like this— so quiet. Y'see? Think of all that emotion that's going on in her mind. I could see it—the school, the friends, will it come out good?—will boys like her?—will she be prettier?—will it hurt?— when will it be?—will it be now, will it be later?

The emotional strain on Mrs. Lubin was unabating. "I wish," she said one day while waiting for Natalie to come out of the recovery room, "I had the money and the time for a little nervous breakdown or a psychiatrist's couch. If my husband was alive I could afford it, but now we are poor and I have to keep going."

A recent "blow" had been Sylvia's announcement that she was quitting college to go to work. (She had just finished her first year on a student loan.) Mrs. Lubin said:

Natalie, who is floundering at 21 to fill in her deprived educational background, was horrified. "What?" she said. "You're leaving school? Do you realize how lucky you are? I wish I had that chance!" And Sylvia yelled at her, "I have to go to work to help bring in an income. Sometimes you have to help somebody else— sometimes a handicapped sister!"

I don't know (Mrs. Lubin sighed) if Sylvia is just looking for a way out because she's so overweight. But if I applied myself and earned more instead of getting frightened and tired and skipping weeks of work while Natalie is recuperating, maybe Sylvia wouldn't feel guilty about staying in school.

A year later, Mrs. Lubin died suddenly of a heart attack. She was 48. "Of course it was a shock," Natalie told me shortly after her mother's death, "but Sylvia and I had to pull ourselves together. There's no use sitting around all day moping. You have to go on with your life, you have to do things." Although they could have moved in with a cousin, the girls chose to remain in their apartment, despite their continuing conflicts. Sylvia had a full-time job as a dental assistant, and Natalie was on social security disability and also babysitting so that she could continue her schooling. "This is what my mother would want me to do, but I would have done it anyway."

Several months later, Natalie had an operation to reshape her nose, with markedly improved results. Though she was far from attractive, the cumulative effect of the numerous operations had sufficiently minimized the grossness of her appearance to allow her to move about in public without attracting undue attention. She dressed more neatly—"I take more care of my clothes and appearance now; before I figured it wouldn't make much difference how I looked." There were other advances as well. She was enrolled full time in college and doing well. "I'm working up to my full potential now," she said. "My mother used to nag me—she was a typical Jewish mother—she'd say 'You're not working up to your potential; if you couldn't do better I wouldn't nag you.' She knew I could do better, but I was always worrying about what others were thinking." Of particular significance, because of the positive psychological implications, was that for the first time Natalie could talk about, retrospectively, the existence of her impediments, and her long-repressed feelings and experiences. Referring to them, she said, "But all this has changed. I am a person all around—mental, physical, everything. I'm walking amongst strangers now—I have a *right* to be among them. Before people weren't willing to accept me. Now I feel part of the group."[6]

[6] While the reality basis for this statement in its entirety might well be questioned, it is Natalie's *perception* of herself and others that is important. The same observation has been made by Dee W. West in his study, "Adaptation to Surgically Induced Facial Disfigurement Among Cancer Patients," unpublished Ph.D. dissertation, University of New York at Buffalo, 1973, p. 239.

As a future worker with handicapped children, with whom she has strong feelings of kinship, Natalie has definite ideas about how they might be helped.

Make them see that even *with* their handicap, they can still do *something* with themselves and not just sit around and become *nothing*. I'd try to bring the best out in them that I can—make them live up to their ability, no more, no less. For example, I know what my abilities are, and I know what they're *not*. And I'd show them that just because they're handicapped doesn't mean that they can't do *anything*.

Parents should not "hover" over their handicapped children. They should treat them normally. Let them do whatever they think they can do, and don't say "You're handicapped; you can't do it" so they'll be discouraged. Let them *try* to do it. Luckily my father did not overprotect me or treat me differently, and my mother was the type—you know—she believed that all children were created *equal*. I mean, some people said, "What did you *do* to her? She's so outgoing and easy to reach." She treated me as if I was normal in every respect. She started with the thought that my sister and I were created equal, which is good. And she did this by treating me as if nothing was *wrong* with me really. I had the normal accidents—scraped knees—you name it, I had it! But she didn't ever bring out, "You're handicapped—you can't do this, you can't do that." And my sister and I were treated exactly alike. When I deserved to be hit, I was hit. When I deserved to be punished, I was punished. And of course when I deserved a reward, I was rewarded. She didn't shelter me from anything.

Teachers, also, should treat the handicapped child the same as other children. Don't set them apart as anything special. Show them that if they're in the school with the other children they have to toe the mark just as anyone else does; [that] they're not going to get away with anything just because they're handicapped. If the child is teased by other children the teacher should not interfere, because right away she'll say, "Look, she's handicapped—let her alone." I'd let the children work it out for themselves, because nine times out of ten the children will eventually become friends. Let them fight their own battles. First of all it's not only not bringing up their handicap, but it will teach them how to cope with people. If the teacher lets well enough alone and doesn't get involved, then it will show the kid he has responsibility and can handle it on his own. He doesn't *need* anybody else. Also, if it shows him he can do something once by himself, then it could open the door.

By a constellation of fortuitous circumstances Natalie, at this writing, is a responsible and self-sufficient young woman.

Her parents' determination to make her feel loved and as capable as other children seems to have provided her with enough ego-strength and tenacity to withstand the searing effects of childhood ostracism. At a critical point in her late adolescence the advanced techniques in plastic surgery offered hope—enough to sustain her from one year to another, while professionals involved in other aspects of her rehabilitation provided assistance and support.

Despite the skepticism and dire predictions of some regarding her "unrealistic ambitions," her defenses permitted her to function, albeit tenuously, and gradually to attempt what others would not dare.

Although Natalie has yet to put her ideas about helping handicapped children into practice (she is still in college and majoring in education), they reveal the extent to which she is coming to terms with her limitations. Denial is gradually giving way to self-acceptance and to a degree of adjustment that no longer verges on the aberrant.

Notes

Selected

Bibliography

Index

Notes

CHAPTER THREE

*1. Revision of pp. 629–638, Macgregor, Frances Cooke, "Some Psychosocial Problems Associated with Facial Deformities," *American Sociological Review*, vol. 16, no. 5, 1951.

*2. Revision of pp. 71–88, Macgregor, Frances Cooke, Theodora M. Abel, Albert Bryt, Edith Lauer, and Serena Weissmann, *Facial Deformities and Plastic Surgery: A Psychosocial Study*, Charles C Thomas, Springfield, Illinois, 1953.

CHAPTER FOUR

*1. Revision of pp. 69–71, 75–81 of Macgregor, et al., *Facial Deformities and Plastic Surgery: A Psychosocial Study*, op. cit.

*2. Revision of pp. 231–233, Macgregor, "Social and Psychological Implications of Dentofacial Disfigurement," *Angle Orthodontist*, vol. 40, no. 3, 1970.

*3. Revision of pp. 125–135, Macgregor, "Social and Cultural Components in the Motivations of Persons Seeking Plastic Surgery of the Nose," *Journal of Health and Social Behavior*, vol. 8, no. 2, 1967.

CHAPTER FIVE

*1. Revision of pp. 37–40, Macgregor, "Psychosocial Approach to Patients with Facial Disfigurement," in *Nursing Care for Plastic Surgery Patients*, edited by Donald Wood-Smith and Pauline Porowski, C. V. Mosby Company, St. Louis, 1967.

CHAPTER SIX

*1. Revision of pp. 3–28, Macgregor, "Social and Psychological Problems Associated with Traumatic Injuries of the Face," in *The Surgical Treatment of Facial Injuries*, third edition, Varaztad H. Kazanjian and John M. Converse, Williams & Wilkins Company, in press.

CHAPTER SEVEN

*1. Revision of pp. 289–292, Macgregor, "Selection of Cosmetic Surgery Patients: Social and Psychological Considerations," *Surgical Clinics of North America: Symposium on Cosmetic Surgery*, edited by Thomas D. Rees, vol. 51, no. 2, W.B. Saunders Company, Philadelphia, 1971.

*2. Revision of p. 126, Macgregor, "Some Psychological Hazards of Plastic Surgery of the Face," *Plastic and Reconstructive Surgery*, vol. 12, no. 2, 1953.

*3. Revision of pp. 292–294, "Selection of Cosmetic Surgery Patients," op. cit.

*4. Revision of pp. 127–129, "Some Psychological Hazards of Plastic Surgery of the Face," op. cit.

*5. Revision of pp. 294–297, "Selection of Cosmetic Surgery Patients," op. cit.

Selected
Bibliography

Abé, Kobo, *The Face of Another*. Alfred A. Knopf, New York, 1966.

Alexander, Chester, "Antipathy and Social Behavior," *American Journal of Sociology*, vol. 51, no. 4, 1946, pp. 288–292.

Allport, Floyd H., *Social Psychology*. Johnson Reprint Corp., New York, 1967.

Allport, Gordon W., *Personality: A Psychological Interpretation*. Henry Holt and Company, New York, 1937.

Allport, Gordon W., and Bernard M. Kramer, "Some Roots of Prejudice," *Journal of Psychology*, vol. 22, 1946, pp. 9–39.

Barker, Roger G., Beatrice A. Wright, Lee Meyerson, and Mollie R. Gonick, *Adjustment to Physical Handicap and Illness: Social Psychology of Physique and Disability*. Social Science Research Council, Bulletin 55, New York, 1953.

Bateson, Gregory, and Margaret Mead, *Balinese Character*. New York Academy of Sciences, New York, 1942.

Birdwhistell, Ray L., *Kinesics and Context: Essays on Body Motion Communication*. University of Pennsylvania Press, Philadelphia, 1970.

Broom, Leonard, Helen P. Beem, and Virginia Harris, "Characteristics of 1,107 Petitioners for Change of Name," *American Sociological Review*, vol. 20, no. 1, 1955, pp. 33–39.

Bryt, Albert, "Psychiatric Aspects," in *Facial Deformities and Plastic Surgery: A Psychosocial Study*, by F. C. Macgregor, et al. Charles C Thomas, Springfield, Illinois, 1953, pp. 166–207.

Burr, Charles W., "Personality and Physiognomy," in *The Human Face: A Symposium*. The Dental Cosmos, Philadelphia, 1935, pp. 81–85.

Callander, John, *Deformities of Dr. Samuel Johnson*, second edition. J. Stockdale and W. Creech, London, 1783.

Clifford, Edward, "Cleft Palate and the Person: Psychological Studies of Its Impact," *Journal of the Southern Medical Association*, vol. 64, no. 12, 1971, pp. 1516–1520.

Cook, Stuart W., "The Judgment of Intelligence from Photographs," *Journal of Abnormal and Social Psychology*, vol. 34, no. 3, 1939, pp. 384–389.

Cooley, Charles H., *Human Nature and the Social Order*. Schocken, New York, 1964.

Davis, Fred, "Deviance Disavowal: The Management of Strained Interaction by the Visibly Handicapped," *Social Problems*, vol. 9, no. 2, 1961, pp. 120–132.

———, *Passage Through Crisis: Polio Victims and Their Families*. Bobbs-Merrill, Indianapolis, 1963.

Ellis, Havelock, *The Soul of Spain*. Houghton Mifflin, Boston, 1931.

Erikson, Erik H., "Identity, Psychosocial," in *International Encyclopedia of the Social Sciences*, vol. 7, 1968, pp. 61–65.

———, *Identity, Youth, and Crisis*. W. W. Norton, New York, 1968.

Friedman, Paul, "The Nose: Some Psychological Reflections," *American Imago*, vol. 8, no. 4, 1951, pp. 3–16.

Goffman, Erving, "Alienation from Interaction," *Human Relations*, vol. 10, no. 1, 1957, pp. 47–60.

———, *Behavior in Public Places*. The Free Press, New York, 1963.

———, "On Face-Work," *Psychiatry: Journal for the Study of Interpersonal Processes*, vol. 18, no. 3, 1955, pp. 213–231.

———, *The Presentation of Self in Everyday Life*. Doubleday, Anchor Books, Garden City, New York, 1959.

———, *Stigma: Notes on the Management of Spoiled Identity*. Prentice-Hall, Englewood Cliffs, New Jersey, 1963.

Gregory, William K., *Our Face from Fish to Man*. G. P. Putnam's Sons, New York, 1929.

Holden, Harold M., *Noses*. World Publishing Company, Cleveland, 1950.

Hooton, Ernest A., *Up from the Ape*, rev. edition. Macmillan Company, New York, 1947.

Huber, Ernst, *Evolution of Facial Musculature and Facial Expression*. The Johns Hopkins Press, Baltimore, 1931.

Huxley, Julian S., and A. C. Haddon, *We Europeans*. Harper and Bros., New York, 1936.

Hviid, Jørgen, *Reactions of the Non-Handicapped Toward the Handicapped*. Gyldendalske Boghandel, Nordisk Forlag A.S., Copenhagen, Denmark, 1972.

Ichheiser, Gustav, "Misunderstandings in Human Relations: A Study in False Social Perception," *American Journal of Sociology*, vol. 55, no. 2, part 2, 1949, pp. 1–70.

———, "The Significance of the Physical Beauty of the Individual in Socio-Psychological and Sociological Explanation," *Zeitschrift für Völkerpsychologie und Soziologie*, September 1928, translated by E. C. Hughes in *An Introduction to Sociology*, revised edition, by Carl A. Dawson and Warner E. Gettys. The Ronald Press Company, New York, 1935, pp. 749–753.

Jacobson, Wayne E., M. T. Edgerton, E. Meyer, A. Canter, and R. Slaughter, "Psychiatric Evaluation of Male Patients Seeking Cosmetic Surgery," *Plastic and Reconstructive Surgery*, vol. 26, no. 4, 1960, pp. 356–372.

Kazanjian, Varaztad H., and John Marquis Converse, *The Surgical Treat-*

ment of Facial Injuries, third edition. Williams & Wilkins Company, Baltimore, in press.

Knorr, Norman J., J. E. Hoopes, and M. T Edgerton, "Psychiatric-Surgical Approach to Adolescent Disturbance in Self Image," *Plastic and Reconstructive Surgery,* vol. 41, no. 3, 1968, pp. 248–253.

Kresky, Beatrice, and Bernard E. Simon, "Infantile Reaction to Facial Disfigurement," *Archives of Surgery,* vol. 82, May 1961, pp. 783–788.

Kutner, Bernard, "Surgeons and Their Patients: A Study in Social Perception," in *Patients, Physicians and Illness,* edited by E. Gartly Jaco. The Free Press, Glencoe, Illinois, 1958, pp. 384–397.

Lauer, Edith, "The Family," in *Facial Deformities and Plastic Surgery: A Psychosocial Study,* by F. C. Macgregor, et al. Charles C Thomas, Springfield, Illinois, 1953, pp. 103–129.

Lavater, Johann Casper, *Physiognomical Bible* (1772), cited by Leo Kanner, "Judging Emotions from Facial Expression," in *Psychological Monographs,* No. 41, Psychological Review Company, Princeton, New Jersey, 1931.

Lewin, Kurt, *Resolving Social Conflicts,* edited by Gertrud W. Lewin. Harper and Bros., New York, 1948.

Linn, Louis, and Irving B. Goldman, "Psychiatric Observations Concerning Rhinoplasty," *Psychosomatic Medicine,* vol. 11, no. 5, 1949, pp. 307–315.

Linton, Ralph, *The Study of Man.* Appleton-Century-Crofts, New York, 1936, 1964.

Lowie, Robert H., *The Crow Indians.* Farrar & Rinehart, New York, 1935.

Macalister, Alexander, "Physiognomy," *Encyclopaedia Britannica,* eleventh edition, vol. 21, 1911, pp. 550–552.

McGinniss, Joe, *The Selling of the President 1968.* Simon and Schuster, New York, 1970.

Macgregor, Frances Cooke, "Psychosocial Approach to Patients with Facial Disfigurement," in *Nursing Care for Plastic Surgery Patients,* edited by Donald Wood-Smith and Pauline Porowski. C. V. Mosby Company, St. Louis, 1967, pp. 35–46.

——, "Selection of Cosmetic Surgery Patients: Social and Psychological Considerations," *Surgical Clinics of North America: Symposium on Cosmetic Surgery,* edited by Thomas D. Rees, vol. 51, no. 2, W. B. Saunders Company, Philadelphia, 1971, pp. 289–298.

——, "Social and Cultural Components in the Motivations of Persons Seeking Plastic Surgery of the Nose," *Journal of Health and Social Behavior,* vol. 8, no. 2, 1967, pp. 125–135.

——, "Social and Psychological Implications of Dentofacial Disfigurement," *Angle Orthodontist,* vol. 40, no. 3, 1970, pp. 231–233.

——, "Social and Psychological Problems Associated with Traumatic Injuries of the Face," in *The Surgical Treatment of Facial Injuries,* third edition, by Varaztad H. Kazanjian and John M. Converse. Williams & Wilkins Company, Baltimore, in press.

——, *Social Science in Nursing: Applications for the Improvement of Patient Care.* Russell Sage Foundation, New York, 1960.

——, "The Sociological Aspects of Facial Deformities," unpublished master's thesis. University of Missouri, 1947.

————, "Some Psychological Hazards of Plastic Surgery of the Face," *Plastic and Reconstructive Surgery*, vol. 12, no. 2, 1953, pp. 123–130.

————, "Some Psycho-social Problems Associated with Facial Deformities," *American Sociological Review*, vol. 16, no. 5, 1951, pp. 629–638.

Macgregor, Frances Cooke, Theodora M. Abel, Albert Bryt, Edith Lauer, and Serena Weissmann, *Facial Deformities and Plastic Surgery: A Psychosocial Study*. Charles C Thomas, Springfield, Illinois, 1953.

Macgregor, Frances Cooke, and Bertram Schaffner, "Screening Patients for Nasal Plastic Operations: Some Sociologic and Psychiatric Considerations," *Psychosomatic Medicine*, vol. 12, no. 5, 1950, pp. 277–291.

Macgregor, Gordon, *Warriors without Weapons*. University of Chicago Press, Chicago, 1946.

Mead, George H., *Mind, Self and Society*. University of Chicago Press, Chicago, 1934.

Mencken, H. L., *The American Language*, fourth edition. Alfred A. Knopf, New York, 1938.

Meyer, Eugene, "Psychiatric Aspects of Plastic Surgery," in *Reconstructive Plastic Surgery*, vol. 1, *General Principles*, edited by John M. Converse. W. B. Saunders Company, Philadelphia, 1964, pp. 365–383.

Meyer, Eugene, "Psychiatric Aspects of Plastic Surgery," in *Reconstruc-Canter*, "Motivational Patterns in Patients Seeking Elective Plastic Surgery: I. Women Who Seek Rhinoplasty," *Psychosomatic Medicine*, vol. 22, no. 3, 1960, pp. 193–201.

Miller, Nathan, *The Child in Primitive Society*. Brentano's, New York, 1928.

Mitford, Jessica, *The American Way of Death*. Fawcett World Library, Crest Books, New York, 1964.

Murphy, Gardner, "Psychological Views of Personality and Contributions to Its Study," in *The Study of Personality: An Interdisciplinary Appraisal*, edited by E. Norbeck, D. Price-Williams, and W. M. McCord. Holt, Rinehart and Winston, New York, 1968, pp. 15–40.

Murphy, Robert F., "Social Distance and the Veil," *American Anthropologist*, vol. 66, no. 6, part I, 1964, pp. 1257–1274.

Opler, Morris E., *An Apache Life-Way*. University of Chicago Press, Chicago, 1941.

Park, Robert E., and Ernest W. Burgess, *Introduction to the Science of Sociology*. University of Chicago Press, Chicago, 1924, 1969; also Heritage of Sociology Series, University of Chicago Press.

Perrin, F. A. C., "Physical Attractiveness and Repulsiveness," *Journal of Experimental Psychology*, vol. 4, June 1921, pp. 203–217.

Pratt, Lois, Arthur Seligman, and George Reader, "Physicians' Views on the Level of Medical Information Among Patients," in *Patients, Physicians and Illness*, edited by E. Gartly Jaco. The Free Press, Glencoe, Illinois, 1958, pp. 222–229.

Reusch, Jurgen, "The Future of Psychologically Oriented Psychiatry," in *Sexuality of Women*, edited by Jules H. Masserman. Grune & Stratton, New York, 1966, pp. 144–163.

Richardson, Stephen A., N. Goodman, A. H. Hastorf, and S. M. Dornbusch, "Cultural Uniformity in Reaction to Physical Disabilities," *American Sociological Review*, vol. 26, no. 2, 1961, pp. 241–247.

Ross, Edward A., *Social Psychology*. Macmillan Company, New York, 1917.

Safilios-Rothschild, Constantina, *The Sociology and Social Psychology of Disability and Rehabilitation*. Random House, New York, 1970.

Savitz, Leonard D., and Richard F. Tomasson, "The Identifiability of Jews," *American Journal of Sociology*, vol. 64, no. 5, 1959, pp. 468–475.

Schilder, Paul, *The Image and Appearance of the Human Body*, Psychological Monographs, No. 4. K. Paul, Trench, Trubner and Company, London, 1935.

Scodel, Alvin, and Harvey Austrin, "The Perception of Jewish Photographs by Non-Jews and Jews," *Journal of Abnormal and Social Psychology*, vol. 54, no. 2, 1957, pp. 278–280.

Seward, Georgene, *Psychotherapy and Culture Conflict*. The Ronald Press, New York, 1956.

Shapiro, Harry L., *The Jewish People: A Biological History*. UNESCO, Paris, 1960.

Simmel, Georg, *Soziologie*. Duncker und Humblot, Leipzig, 1908.

Simon, William, and John H. Gagnon, "Homosexuality: The Formulation of a Sociological Perspective," *Journal of Health and Social Behavior*, vol. 8, no. 3, 1967, pp. 177–185.

Stonequist, Everett V., *The Marginal Man: A Study in Personality and Culture Conflict*. Charles Scribner's Sons, New York, 1937.

The Structure of Attitudes Toward the Disabled, Brief. Division of Research and Demonstration Grants, Social and Rehabilitation Service, Department of Health, Education, and Welfare, Washington, D.C., vol. 4, no. 6, December 15, 1970.

Thorek, Max, *The Face in Health and Disease*. F. A. Davis and Company, Philadelphia, 1946.

Tiet, James A., "Tattooing and Face and Body Painting of the Thompson Indians, British Columbia," in *Forty-Fifth Annual Report of the Bureau of American Ethnology*. U.S. Government Printing Office, Washington, D.C., 1930, pp. 403–439.

Updegraff, Howard L., and Karl A. Menninger, "Some Psychoanalytic Aspects of Plastic Surgery," *American Journal of Surgery*, vol. 25, September 1934, pp. 554–558.

Viscardi, Jr., Henry, *A Man's Stature*. John Day Company, New York, 1952.

Webb, Mary, *Precious Bane*. E. P. Dutton & Co., New York, 1926, and Random House, The Modern Library, New York, undated.

West, Dee W., "Adaptation to Surgically Induced Facial Disfigurement Among Cancer Patients," unpublished Ph.D. dissertation. University of New York at Buffalo, 1973.

Wirth, Lewis, *The Ghetto*. University of Chicago Press, Chicago, 1928.

Wolfenstein, Martha, "Two Types of Jewish Mothers," in *Childhood in Contemporary Cultures*, edited by Margaret Mead and Martha Wolfenstein. University of Chicago Press, Chicago, 1955, pp. 424–440.

Wright, Beatrice A., *Physical Disability—A Psychological Approach*. Harper and Bros., New York, 1960.

Wyckoff, Gene, *The Image Makers*. The Macmillan Company, New York, 1968.

Index of Names

Index of Subjects